I'M TOO YOUNG TO HAVE BREAST CANCER!

I'M TOO YOUNG TO HAVE BREAST CANCER!

Regain Control of Your Life, Career,
Family, Sexuality, and Faith

BETH LEIBSON-HAWKINS

LifeLine
Press

A Regnery Publishing Company, Washington, D.C.

Library of Congress Cataloging-in-Publication Data

Leibson-Hawkins, Beth.
 I'm too young to have breast cancer! : regain control of your life, career, family, sexuality, and faith / Beth Leibson-Hawkins.
   p. cm.
 Includes index.
 ISBN 0-89526-055-7
 1. Breast—Cancer—Popular works. 2. Young women—Diseases—Popular works. I. Title.
 RC280.B8L355 2004
 616.99'449—dc22
               2004017498

Published in the United States by
LifeLine Press
A Regnery Publishing Company
One Massachusetts Avenue NW
Washington, DC 20001

Visit us at www.lifelinepress.com

Distributed to the trade by
National Book Network
4501 Forbes Boulevard, Suite 200
Lanham, MD 20706
Printed on acid-free paper
Manufactured in the United States of America

10 9 8 7 6 5 4 3 2 1

Books are available in quantity for promotional or premium use. Write to Director of Special Sales, Regnery Publishing, Inc., One Massachusetts Avenue NW, Washington, DC 20001, for information on discounts and terms or call (202) 216-0600.

To my beloved Robert, my darlings Maya and Ari,
and my dear friend Darcy

❧ Contents ❧

How I Came to Write This Book

I hadn't heard from Roberta in ages. We kept in touch for a number of years, despite several moves, and I had always been impressed by her intelligence, her drive, and her lively sense of humor. Though she grew up in Connecticut, Roberta always struck me as a true New Yorker: straightforward and businesslike, but with heart.

AFTER A SIX-MONTH LAPSE IN OUR CORRESPONDENCE, I was stunned to read her e-mail: "Sorry I've been out of touch; I was diagnosed with breast cancer a few months ago and had a lumpectomy and then a mastectomy. I am currently on chemo . . ."

Wait a minute. Breast cancer? But Roberta was twenty-seven years old. I thought breast cancer struck only older women.

My head was spinning. I couldn't make the connection between Roberta's age and her diagnosis. Roberta was in great health; she never got sick, barely even got the sniffles. She jogged regularly, watched what she ate, drank in moderation, and didn't smoke. She couldn't have breast cancer.

I was wrong.

⟡

According to the National Cancer Institute, breast cancer is the leading cause of cancer mortality in women under age thirty-five.

Roberta's diagnosis terrified me. I am five years older than she; if she was vulnerable to breast cancer, I was even more so. That night, I did a manual breast exam, but didn't trust my own checking. I went in a month or two early for my regular gynecologic exam, explaining that I wanted the doctor to check my breasts. (I was fine.) Two months later, when I saw my internist for a flu shot, I had her check my breasts, just in case. (Still fine.) And breast self-exams, which I used to do sporadically, are now a regularly scheduled activity.

As Roberta described her illness—the lessons she learned as well as her struggles and frustrations—I tried to figure out what I could do. She mentioned that she couldn't find any books about dealing with breast cancer as a young woman. To learn how other women had made decisions, Roberta got names from her doctors and phoned complete strangers to ask about their experiences.

Well, there it was: I'd find her a book about young breast cancer survivors. That couldn't be difficult, I thought. With thousands of young women diagnosed annually, I *knew* there had to be a book aimed at them, their family, and friends. Not a medical text, but a collection of intimate conversations between survivors and readers. I just knew such a book was out there.

Again, I was wrong.

I searched bookstores and cruised the Internet, but I couldn't find a book that would help Roberta feel less alone. There is a lot of medical information and even a good amount of psychosocial material on breast cancer in general. I found a number of books about women in their fifties and sixties and some that spoke to the concerns of breast cancer survivors of all ages. But I couldn't find a single volume devoted to women diagnosed at or before age forty, the age at which doctors recommend women have a baseline mammogram (the test that can find cancer well before a lump appears).

"You could write a book about young women with breast cancer," Roberta proposed when my family and I met her for a late breakfast in a deli near her Manhattan apartment. It was a "chemo weekend," about four months into treatment, and Roberta scarcely touched her buttered bagel. I felt guilty about my spinach omelet.

"But I don't know anything about breast cancer," I protested.

"Neither did I before I was diagnosed," she said. "You could learn as easily as I did. Start with *Dr. Susan Love's Breast Book.*" She took a sip of hot tea. "You're a writer," she reminded me. "And you're interested in women's health issues."

I didn't know what to say. I looked at Roberta's greenish complexion, her thinning hair, accented with a touch of gray that she couldn't dye during treatment. "Of course," I said. "Of course I can write a book about breast cancer."

And so I began. First, I perused books and medical journals. I was quickly overwhelmed by the enormity of the task. I kept thinking that if it was difficult for me to find information, it must be even harder and more stressful for someone dealing with the fear and anger that follows a cancer diagnosis.

I put together a series of questions and began to look for survivors. I had to find women who were interested in sharing their stories with a complete stranger who had no personal experience with breast cancer. I worked with hospitals, support groups, and other health care organizations. I posted signs (enlisting friends in the effort) and contacted everyone I knew. People were kind enough to pass my request along; one woman I spoke with said that my request had come to her via Santiago, Chile.

I found a wide range of women. They live all over the country, in urban, suburban, and rural settings. Some have a life partner, others live alone; some have children, others do not. They have different ethnic and religious backgrounds and sexual orientations. They represent a range of socioeconomic levels, from waitress to attorney, from factory worker to college administrator. With one exception, they all received their diagnoses and treatments over the past ten years. Jacquie, whose story appears in the "Pregnancy, Children, and Family" chapter, was diagnosed in the mid-1980s. The treatments these women received, especially chemotherapy, were based on what was available at the time.

I was continually surprised by the graciousness of the women I contacted. While I was overcome by the emotion of their stories, I was also inspired. I am immensely grateful to the women who volunteered to share their experiences with me, who were willing—and often thrilled—to talk with me for hours and answer my seemingly endless questions.

This is not a medical book. It does not address choosing a doctor, understanding a diagnosis, or selecting from among treatment options. Instead, it focuses on issues of day-to-day life.

Being diagnosed with a life-threatening disease is often a terrifying experience that pervades every aspect of life, from work to sexuality to family to spirituality. Most older breast cancer survivors worry about whether—or how—to make changes in well-established careers. They consider how their diagnosis will affect their grown children, especially grown daughters. They may even worry about how to break the news to their grandchildren.

The experiences and concerns of women who are diagnosed with breast cancer in their twenties and thirties are much different. Studies show that younger breast cancer patients report higher levels of emotional distress than older women with the disease, and that young breast cancer survivors have a more difficult time recuperating emotionally than middle-aged and older survivors. Researchers also suggest that women ages forty and younger have a greater fear of death, more concerns about work and career, and increased worries about the effects on their families and lost opportunities for childbearing. One study found that significantly more older breast cancer patients considered themselves "mostly happy" than did younger ones.

Researchers provide a number of reasons for this increased difficulty. Younger breast cancer survivors often have less emotional and logistical support than women who have more established social and professional lives. Sometimes they have plenty of friends and relatives willing and able to help them, but they just don't know how to ask for help or they feel that they ought to be able to "go it alone."

Also, part of the challenge is societal. Women in their twenties and thirties aren't supposed to have life-threatening illnesses. Early adulthood is a time for beginnings, for exploration, for self-definition. Not for cancer.

The "why me?" factor is far greater at twenty-seven than at seventy. Jacquie explained that when she was diagnosed, it didn't matter that she was a woman and it didn't matter that she was African American. The only relevant fact was that she was twenty-nine years old. Paulette, who found her lump at age twenty-six, agreed; she remembers brushing off a Reach for Recovery volunteer in the hospital because of the age difference. "When you're twenty-something or in your early thirties," she said, it's hard to listen when "you're looking at somebody who lived a lot longer than you before getting the disease."

Nor are peers ready to be faced with such overt proof of their own mortality. Younger people—breast cancer survivors and others—have greater expectations of their physical health than older people. Because fear sometimes outweighs sympathy, the young breast cancer survivor is often more alone than the older patient. Nora talks about a boyfriend who broke up with her because he couldn't face the thought of losing her to cancer; he would rather end the relationship on his own timetable. And Helen, Becky, and Nora all had friends who just weren't available when they were most needed.

As I interviewed these young breast cancer survivors, five areas of concern kept surfacing over and over: regaining control of their lives; work and career; sexuality and dating; family and children; and spirituality. These aspects of life have nothing to do with medicine, treatment, or mortality, but they seemed to be the most important to these young women.

It is part of human nature to assume that we will maintain the same level of control over our lives today as we had yesterday. But when a woman is diagnosed with breast cancer, this is no longer the case. Some women feel that their bodies have betrayed them, that they have lost control over their lives. In "Regaining Control," there are women who successfully did just that; some by managing every facet of their lives carefully and thoroughly, some by focusing on one major goal at a time.

"Work and Career" profiles women who found that their breast cancer made them reevaluate their career priorities. For some, soul-searching led to a radical change in career direction. Others found that they were eager to return to the jobs they had and the careers they had been building, reaffirming for them that their original career choices had been right. Still others chose to change their work/life balance. One woman elected to switch to a less demanding job and to physically remove herself from the workplace environment by going to a vacation house on the weekends.

Dating during breast cancer treatment and afterward can be a frightening prospect. Researchers report that younger breast cancer survivors have more problems with self-esteem, feminine self-image, and intimacy than older survivors. Women may be anxious about a date's response to a missing or reconstructed breast or to hair loss or weight gain. The women profiled in "Sexuality and Dating" felt burnt (by radiation), scarred (from surgery), and generally undesirable. Each struggled with regaining a sense of her own sexuality. One woman was greatly helped by undergoing breast reconstruction, whereas one athletic woman decided against it, for very personal reasons. Another met a man while she was undergoing treatment, started dating him once she was finished, and married him two years after her diagnosis.

Women with young children already juggle multiple roles. Add breast cancer and the balancing act becomes even more precarious. In addition, there are questions of how to discuss the disease—and mortality—with young children. In "Pregnancy, Children, and Family," there are women who have struggled with and continue to worry about these issues. Another major decision is whether to have children, given the potential for increased risk of cancer recurrence that may stem from the hormonal surges of pregnancy. Right in the middle of their childbearing years, these young women found themselves facing an unexpected range of challenges and choices.

Faith often gives us strength. Yet coming face-to-face with one's own mortality at such a young age can deal a devastating blow to one's spirituality. Issues of faith and spiritual belief became paramount to the women profiled in "Faith, Religion, and Spirituality." One turned to religion in her critical time of struggle, creating religious ceremonies to say goodbye to her breast and to embrace her life. Another left the religion of her childhood and turned to another because she found it provided more meaningful answers. Still another decided that her spirituality was more about raising and considering questions than believing in anything in particular. She felt that the very process of reconsidering one's life and goals—a process often spurred by a life-threatening disease and one that nearly every woman in this book has undertaken—is essentially a spiritual journey.

❧

The sixteen voices in this book demonstrate that young women can—and do—live with and through breast cancer, and triumph over it in ways that profoundly surprise them. For one woman, diagnosed at age thirty-two, running the New York City Marathon seven months after completing treatment was her symbol of conquering the illness. Having breast cancer helped another woman see that she is stronger and more confident than she had thought. And as Roberta told me: "There is life after breast cancer—life without boobs—and often it is a much better life."

❧

I have written this book for the nearly quarter of a million young American women age forty and under who were diagnosed with breast cancer. They know that not every face of breast cancer has laugh lines and graying hair. That not every survivor has a solid career, a long-term partner, grown children, and an established life.

Despite the number of young women who live with the disease, there are relatively few resources geared toward them. The women I interviewed told me they felt lonely after their diagnoses. One twenty-six-year-old went to the bookstores and found plenty of information on breast cancer, but nothing that spoke to her as a young woman. When such a young woman is diagnosed with breast cancer, it doesn't matter that she is a woman, it doesn't matter that she is African American or Korean or Caucasian or Hispanic or Buddhist or Jewish or Catholic or Republican or Democratic or Independent. The only relevant fact is that she is only twenty-six years old.

People find it difficult to believe that breast cancer can hit women so young. Young bodies are supposed to be strong. They're not supposed to get sick. It is difficult to equate an otherwise healthy-looking twenty- or thirty-something with the word "cancer." So we as a society—from doctors and nurses to public policy makers and social workers—often fail to provide enough help. Many young women concerned about a lump in their breast often hear, from their own health care providers, that they are "too young to worry about cancer."

But these medical professionals are wrong. A woman has a one in seven chance of developing breast cancer during her lifetime. That possibility increases with age, yes, but this statistic does not imply that young women are somehow invulnerable. More than 11,000 women under age 40 will be diagnosed with breast cancer this year and close to 1,300 will die, according to the Young Survival Coalition. Currently, in the United States alone, nearly 250,000 women under age 40 are living with breast cancer, according to the coalition.

This book tells the stories of women who are "too young to have breast cancer."

※〜 Chapter One 〜※

Regaining Control

*Nora found it hard to believe that she couldn't just go to
the drugstore, spend twelve bucks, and be better in a week.*

WHEN A WOMAN IS DIAGNOSED WITH BREAST CANCER, her life
choices narrow from a panorama to a pinhole. Her ability to make
choices, to be in control, has seemingly disappeared. This is particularly a concern for young women, who are making major life choices
and establishing long-term patterns.

Many young women who have battled breast cancer feel as though
their bodies have betrayed them. They naturally assumed they could
count on their health, especially if they ate well and exercised regularly. They thought serious illness—particularly cancer—was a concern for later in life.

Roberta coped with breast cancer by applying her management
skills to every facet of her life. She orchestrated her treatment and
created a system of rewards for every time she had chemotherapy. She
deftly managed her career; her first action after diagnosis was to

1

install an extra phone line in her apartment so she could work from home. She controlled the flow of personal information to family and friends by setting up one phone tree among her friends and another for her relatives. And she deliberately scheduled in social time between medical appointments and recuperation time.

Lanita's greatest concern was to regain control over her body, to feel at home again in the body that betrayed her. To achieve this larger goal, she set herself a series of smaller challenges: get to the kitchen counter, reach the coffee mugs in the cabinet, run the New York City Marathon all the way to the end. Lanita was not an extremely athletic woman; she ran for personal pleasure and challenge, rather than out of a strong competitive urge. But setting and meeting physical challenges to regain control of her life was critical to her recovery.

HOW DO I REGAIN CONTROL OF MY LIFE?

꿏ⵋ Roberta, 27: The Patient as Manager

TWENTY-SEVEN-YEAR-OLD ROBERTA spent Mondays through Thursdays on the road, working upwards of sixty hours a week; she typically earned two hundred thousand frequent-flier miles a year. Her background was in public health, but her consulting assignments had more to do with the business end of managing major hospitals and medical schools. Roberta enjoyed her job immensely, from interviewing staff to analyzing piles of data. She was highly organized, constantly compiling lists and checking off completed tasks.

Tall and slender, with walnut eyes and thick, dark brown, shoulder-length hair, Roberta played hard, too. When she came home to New York City after long days on the road, she partied with her friends, bar hopped, went to the theater, and—inevitably—did a little work on her laptop. In her spare time, Roberta ran two to three miles several times a week.

Family was very important to Roberta. Her mother, Pat, took the train in from Connecticut regularly for afternoon shopping sprees. They chatted frequently on the phone and even vacationed together.

Roberta shared her two-bedroom apartment, located in a trendy lower Manhattan neighborhood just blocks from New York City's South Street Seaport, with her eighty-five-year-old uncle. The low-key conversations between the two balanced out Roberta's high-energy work and social lives. After long trips away, she looked forward to catching up with Uncle Lou over a cup of steaming Earl Grey. Their nineteenth-floor apartment represented an interesting combination of twenty-something and octogenarian. The living room was organized, sedate, and functional; the stereo was a recent addition, and only the wine-red sofa hinted at Roberta's exuberance. Mezuzot marked the doorposts, in keeping with Jewish tradition, and the balcony offered a magnificent view of the city's skyline.

Somehow Roberta juggled a high-powered career, regular exercise, a busy social calendar, a strong connection to her family, and a commitment to Judaism. She maintained that delicate balance among commitments by making lists, sleeping five hours a night, and being a manager *par excellence*. Roberta was a woman in control of her life.

Breast cancer changed all that.

Playing It Safe

Roberta discovered her cancer when she went for her annual physical. All the test results were normal, except the Pap smear and urine culture. The doctor told her not to worry. He had seen this "postmenstrual result" before and recommended she come back in six months.

Roberta was a little nervous about the abnormal Pap smear. She decided not to wait half a year and made an appointment with a gynecologist a few weeks later. The gynecologist said that the Pap smear looked completely normal. He also performed a routine breast exam.

"By the way," he asked, "did you know you have a lump in your breast?"

The lump was movable and very small. It was under her left arm and Roberta could barely locate it.

"It's probably a benign fibroadenoma, not uncommon among women in their teens and twenties," the gynecologist said. "But why don't you play it safe," he suggested. "Why don't you go see a breast surgeon to have it checked out? Preferably in the next two weeks." He sounded calm, but Roberta wasn't quite convinced. After all, what had started out as a routine physical, a single appointment with her general practitioner, had already expanded to a series of visits with specialists. She shared her thoughts with her mother, who asked to join her when she went to see the breast surgeon.

After the examination, the surgeon talked about unrelated topics, mentioning his own daughter and noting Roberta's close relationship with Pat. Almost as an aside, he said, "By the way, you have a fibroadenoma and I'd like to remove it."

"I don't believe in unnecessary surgery," Roberta responded quickly.

The doctor explained that he was sure the lump was benign, but wanted to take it out because it might grow and her breast would become strangely shaped. Roberta was still unsure, but eventually she agreed to the surgery. They set an appointment for the following month. But then Roberta looked over at her mother, sitting across the room, quietly digging her nails into her hands. Roberta rescheduled the appointment for the next Monday.

＊✿＊

When they chatted on the phone that evening, Roberta's best friend, Stella, picked up on the fear in Roberta's voice. "I want you to fly here, to Boston, this weekend," Stella said. "I'm getting you a ticket. Get on the plane."

The two had been friends for eight years; they had met in college, while studying in England. Roberta liked Stella because her friend always managed to take her mind off serious things. That weekend was a prime example. They partied on Friday night and again on Saturday night. Stella kept introducing Roberta to friends, trying to set her up with dates. For most of the weekend, Roberta wasn't thinking about Monday morning.

That Saturday night, at about two o'clock, after hours of club hopping, they talked about the biopsy. "I don't want to do this," Roberta said.

"You have to," her friend responded. "You have to take it out."

"What if something's wrong?" Roberta countered.

"You Said It Was Nothing"

When she emerged from the biopsy, Roberta felt fine.

"Hey, Mom, look at me! The anesthesia was great."

"That's wonderful, honey," Pat said, trying to smile. "Are you up for some lunch? And then the doctor wants to see you in his office." Roberta was surprised that the doctor wanted to see her so quickly.

Mother and daughter went to a nearby restaurant and discussed Roberta's current consulting project over grilled cheese sandwiches and french fries. When they walked into the doctor's office and sat down, Pat gripped Roberta's hand tightly. The doctor looked at Roberta.

"You have breast cancer," he began.

Roberta laughed. "That's really funny."

"You have breast cancer," the doctor said.

"Come on—quit joking with me," she said. "You said it was nothing. You did a great job with the scar."

"You have breast cancer," he repeated.

Roberta looked at her mother, who sat staring into space. Not crying, not saying anything.

"What does that mean?" Roberta asked.

"We don't know yet," the surgeon said.

Roberta felt lost and dazed; she would later learn that this feeling was a common response to a diagnosis of breast cancer. "I need to know what I have to do."

"You're not ready for that," the surgeon said.

"Don't tell me what I'm ready for and what I'm not ready for," Roberta said firmly, trying to regain some of the control she felt quickly slipping through her fingers. "Just talk to me about what I have to do."

The surgeon explained that she had two options: lumpectomy and radiation, or mastectomy. Roberta knew what a mastectomy was. But suddenly, this was different. They weren't discussing a general condition or even a patient at one of her client hospitals. This was *her* breast.

When she got home, she could remember little of the conversation. She was surprised by that—she usually had an excellent memory— but was glad that her mother had come to the appointment, to keep track of all the details. She worried that losing her ability to retain details was a sign that she was losing control and would hamper her capacity to manage this new situation.

Late that night, Roberta was wide awake, unable to sleep. She went out into the living room and woke up her mother, who had been napping on the couch.

For the first time, she said the words out loud. "I've got cancer."

Both Roberta and Pat broke down. They cried and held on to each other very tightly.

"How am I going to make it?" Roberta asked.

"You've got to," Pat responded. "You're my only daughter. You're going to be fine. We'll face this. Together."

Sharing the News

For Roberta, the worst part was waiting, not knowing what to tell friends and family. She wanted their support, but didn't feel she could tell people the news until she had the complete story. She wanted to be able to get on the phone and say "I'll be okay." But, for the first time in her life, Roberta couldn't say "I'm fine, no big deal."

By the time Roberta finished the five-day marathon of doctors' appointments, her mother and stepfather had contacted everyone in the family. All the out-of-towners were headed to New York. Roberta felt that she wasn't ready for that many sympathetic faces and told Pat to stop all the plans; she wanted to be alone.

Uncle Lou was safe; Roberta knew he wouldn't overwhelm her with emotion. In fact, as the months went on, the words "breast cancer" never came out of his mouth, at least not around Roberta. It was comforting to know there was one person would never break down in tears in front of her.

Taking Control

Roberta knew she couldn't control the cancer, couldn't influence how it would respond to treatment. But she knew she could damn well engineer the logistics of her care.

She responded just as she would to a consulting assignment. She made a list of people to call and set herself a series of goals to reach by the end of each day. She was going to get this cancer thing squared away as quickly as possible and get back to her career. Her first step was to call the telephone company and order an extra phone line; that would allow her to work from home.

Next, Roberta called her office and said she needed to stop working on the current project, effective immediately. "I need six weeks to two months off," she said. "I'm having surgery and I don't know when I'll be back." The staffing coordinator was silent. Dropping out mid-project was unheard of. But then again, so was Roberta being sick.

She called her two mentors at the consulting firm and explained the situation. "You name it," both said, "and you'll get it."

"I need two months off altogether." Roberta began listing specifics. "Then I need an easy assignment in New York City for about six months," she said. "Beyond that, I'm not sure; I need to take some time to think about all this."

Within an hour, new staff was assigned to the Florida project and Roberta was granted a two-month leave of absence. One of the partners in the firm approached all of Roberta's friends in the company and offered them time off to help her.

Once Roberta began sharing her news, support poured in from friends and family. Cards, balloons, flowers, phone calls. And piles and piles of hats: baseball caps, floppy felt hats, oversize sun bonnets. Roberta's favorite was a black floppy hat with a big black bow. She had seen it and loved it, but thought it was too expensive. Friends bought it and sent it to her.

Roberta was overwhelmed by the number of people who called to check on her. She set up a screening system that spared her having to repeat her story endlessly. She would say to friends, "I'm going to tell you some news and when we get off the phone, I want you to call your mother or your best friend." Everyone needed help to handle the news. She would keep her mother and her five "cheerleaders" up to date on all developments, and everyone else, including colleagues, would contact these people. Pat kept in touch with the relatives.

Everyone responded to Roberta's emotional state. If she cried, her friends, relatives, and colleagues would cry; if she got flustered, they got flustered. She realized she had to stay calm and act as though everything was going to be all right. That way, everybody fed off her positive energy, which, in turn, kept her spirits up.

Lumpectomy or Mastectomy?

Roberta's doctors disagreed on the proper course of treatment. One breast surgeon told her to have a mastectomy. The second recommended a lumpectomy, saying there was no reason to have a mastectomy. A third doctor said, "You're a big girl, do whatever you want." Roberta was very frustrated. She had thought her doctors' superior medical knowledge and experience would guide her decisions.

Fortunately, her health care background helped. She realized that there's a different language to breast cancer and that she had to learn the lingo. She brought the skills she honed in her consulting work—researching, making decisions, and taking charge—to her battle against breast cancer.

She read a great deal and talked to lots of people. The first decision was the hardest: lumpectomy or mastectomy? She stood on the balcony of her nineteenth-story apartment and looked up at the Manhattan skyline. She realized that there was little difference in survival statistics between the two operations, particularly given the results of her pathology report. Should she go with a mastectomy for peace of mind? Or should she go with a lumpectomy and keep her breast?

She decided to follow her gut. She wanted a lumpectomy. If she was going to lose a breast, she wanted to be sure that it was absolutely necessary, not just preventive. Once she made the decision, she felt as though a huge weight had been lifted from her shoulders.

A Regular Person

The surgeon warned Roberta that she would be out of commission for two to three weeks after surgery. But she was determined to leave the hospital as soon as possible. She spent just one night in the hospital and was back at work two days after the operation, with minimal side effects.

But the margins weren't clean; the lumpectomy failed to remove all of the cancerous cells. Roberta was left with the same two options to deal with the cancer still in her breast: lumpectomy and radiation, or mastectomy. Her surgeon recommended mastectomy.

"I'm having a party," Stella said. "Why don't you come?"

"I'm recovering from surgery," Roberta said, thinking her friend was nuts. "And I'm in New York."

"So what?" Stella countered, then hung up. She called back ten minutes later, saying, "I've got a ride to Boston for you. He's picking you up in two hours. He's cute and he's Jewish." So Roberta found herself at a party the weekend after her lumpectomy, toting a huge ice pack on her arm to ease the pain in the muscles that had been damaged. A friend stood at her side so no one would bump into her.

She tried to mingle, but finally decided that she needed a fluffy pillow more than anything else. "I'm going back to your place. It's midnight and I'm really tired," Roberta told Stella.

"No," Stella responded. "We're going dancing."

They stayed out dancing until four o'clock in the morning. At the time, Roberta couldn't figure out what Stella was doing. But later on, she realized that Stella didn't treat her like a cancer patient. She treated her like a regular person.

A Marginal Decision

When she got back to New York, Roberta had an appointment with her breast surgeon to have her stitches removed.

"So, what are you going to do about the unclean margins?" he asked. "You've got to do it soon." They discussed the details of her choices again. Then the doctor added, "You should have done a mastectomy in the first place. I recommended that before."

That was the point, Roberta later realized, when she should have changed doctors. Her body was giving her enough pressure—she didn't need additional stress from an unsupportive physician.

Lumpectomy or mastectomy, lumpectomy or mastectomy. Once again, Roberta turned the possibilities over and over in her mind. "I drove myself crazy," she remembers. She talked to friends, fellow survivors, even the plastic surgeon, who had figured he would never hear from her after she decided on a lumpectomy. She worried about whether a man would want her, would want damaged goods. She worried about what sex would be like without feeling in her breast.

She wished it were an easier decision. She almost wished she'd had a huge tumor and *had* to have a mastectomy. She couldn't believe that she had to make such a difficult decision twice.

Roberta decided she didn't want to be faced with this choice a third time. She figured if God had wanted the lumpectomy to work, it would have worked the first time. She decided to undergo the mastectomy.

The second operation was more painful than the first, but Roberta still bounced back more quickly than the two months her doctors had predicted. She spent just two nights in the hospital, taking painkillers most of the time. When she returned home, she took pain medication for a few more days, and then began working from home. She returned to the office within a week, dismantling her home office far ahead of schedule. She pelted her surgeon with questions: How much can I bench-press now? Should I get a flu shot? Can I wear underwire bras?

꒰꒱

The loss of a breast—the impact on her sexuality—was a big issue for Roberta. She was sure that no one would ever want to touch her. She was certain she could never change in a gym again. Roberta wanted to feel whole again, so she decided to have breast reconstruction. Though she realized that not being lopsided would make it easier to dress and easier to regain a sense of balance, she chose reconstruction for psychological reasons. She knew she would have no feeling in the reconstructed breast. "It's simply vanity," she explained to friends and family.

Reconstruction was the most painful surgical procedure Roberta experienced. But it was worth it. She joked with her plastic surgeon: "I hope you did a good job. I plan to put a lot of wear and tear on this thing."

Roberta's friends helped her come to terms with her new breast. One male friend jokingly offered to try it out. But perhaps even more important was a new boyfriend, a man who saw her fight against breast cancer as evidence of strength, not weakness.

Chemotherapy Means No Chocolate?

Roberta began a course of chemotherapy that would last for six months. Those were six hard months. Roberta felt she lost all control of her body—vomiting, constipation, diarrhea, hair falling out, skin turning white, black veins, bags under her eyes. She had no power over anything—over making a pimple go away or getting feeling back in her arm. Her body dictated what she could and could not do, how she could and could not act, what she could and could not eat. To add to her sense of powerlessness, chemotherapy patients receive a seemingly endless list of rules: no chocolate, no sunbathing, no sushi, no alcohol, plenty of liquids.

Roberta realized that staying alive meant maintaining some semblance of her pre-cancer life. So, even on chemo weekends, she went to bars with friends. She figured she was going to throw up no matter what she did, so she might as well go out and see people. "I'm not very good at staying home and being bored," she said. She brightened her normally black wardrobe with reds and purples and carried an extra-large pocketbook. The bag bulged with makeup (to give some color to her now paper-white skin) and a plastic container (to hide the odor of vomit, in case she couldn't make it to the bathroom in time). When she got to the bar, Roberta sipped soft drinks instead of alcohol.

Roberta was tired, really tired, a particularly challenging symptom for a woman who previously thought of sleep as an occasional hobby. She never thought anything could tire her out so much she would sleep thirteen hours a night. But during chemo, she took a blanket and pillow to work for afternoon naps. Her once marathon days were cut in half.

Rewards worked as encouragement. Every time Roberta had a chemo treatment, she bought herself a treat to fix up her room: a CD rack one month, a small TV table the next. She figured that chemo was the most awful experience she would ever go through. If she was going to do it, she decided, she was going to buy something expensive every single time.

Seeking Support

During her chemotherapy treatments, Roberta realized that, despite the support of her friends and family, she needed to establish ties with other young breast cancer survivors. She knew she needed to talk to women who had had breast cancer, women her own age. She wanted to know she wasn't alone, that other people understood what she was feeling. She selected a formal support group specifically for women in their twenties and thirties, but she was still the youngest by five or six years; somehow the chemistry wasn't right. She left that group and began to meet regularly with other young cancer survivors she had met through her job, through her doctors, and at the formal support group—all women she'd bonded with. Every couple of weeks, the women had dinner and shared stories and concerns, triumphs and terrors. They talked about lack of metastasis, unclean margins, recurrences, and implants.

Even though Uncle Lou wasn't a sounding board for Roberta, living with him was comfortable. They would sit on the red couch, sip tea, and talk. Sometimes, if she tried to wash the dishes, he would say, "You're not supposed to do that, you're sick." Occasionally, when she couldn't get up from the couch on her own, he would offer a hand. Other times, he would take a fatherly tone and tell her, "I think you

Survivor Suggestions on Support Groups and Systems

▢ Try to find a support group; there are plenty of groups focusing on young survivors these days (see Resources on page 255).

▢ If you can't find a support group of young women, try to make connections in the group that is available.

▢ Remember, there are support groups to address other issues, such as single parenting.

▢ If you cannot find a support group that works for you, try to create your own network of support.

▢ If support groups begin to make it more complicated or painful, stop going to the meetings.

▢ Find a mentor who can be your support and your friend. Find someone to confide in.

▢ Remember that people bring different life experiences to a breast cancer diagnosis; knowing that people cope with their concerns in differing ways may help you handle it.

ought to go to bed." But he never made too big a deal of it, always treating her like his niece, not his *sick* niece.

"It's Just a Breast"

Roberta wanted to take charge of her doctors, too. She began thinking about her surgeon's awkward bedside manner. He was an excellent surgeon and had plenty of experience treating the disease. But he and Roberta never connected on a personal level. And that was going to be a problem if he was going to check her every six months for five years, and then annually for the rest of her life. She didn't appreciate his reluctance to answer her many specific questions. She was still bothered that he told her, "It's just a breast" when recommending a mastectomy. She eventually came to agree, but she needed to figure that out on her own. As she told her mother, "A woman is going to understand why losing your breast is a big deal, whereas the only way to explain it to a man is to say, 'How would you feel if I chopped off your testicles?'"

At the same time, Roberta felt a certain loyalty to this man who had diagnosed and removed her cancer, the man who literally saved her life.

She thought about her other doctors, whom she liked. Whenever Roberta asked a question, her oncologist would tell her not to rush into decisions, saying, "Not too quick. Call me, e-mail me. Take your time." Her plastic surgeon, too, seemed to understand the emotional importance of breasts; he grasped that it was important for the breast to look and feel as normal as he could make it. She wanted to like her breast surgeon, too.

But it took a while for Roberta the manager to take over from Roberta the breast cancer patient. It wasn't until she finished with all her surgery and was well into chemotherapy that she decided it was time to find a new breast surgeon.

She approached her search with characteristic thoroughness. She collected opinions and advice from relatives, friends, friends of friends, and her other doctors. When she interviewed doctors, she inquired about everything from waiting time, to how often they talk to the average patient, to who was on call on weekends and holidays. It was worth it, Roberta decided, to take the time to pick the right physician, to regain control over that aspect of treatment.

A Man's Touch

One evening, Roberta's friend Russell asked her to meet him at a bar. She had just finished a round of chemotherapy and wasn't feeling up to it; she just wanted to stay home where she could get sick in a dignified manner. Russell persisted, saying there was someone he wanted her to meet. Finally, Roberta agreed and went out to see Russell. She felt miserable the whole night. The next day, she barely remembered where she'd been, much less meeting Lee, the man Russell had brought with him.

When Lee called her the following night, Roberta didn't even recognize his name. When he invited her out for a drink, she was baffled. Didn't he know she had cancer? She couldn't date! They talked on the phone for two hours, making plans to get together a few days later, along with Russell. She told him she wouldn't go out with him unless there were at least two other people present. She wanted to make sure that absolutely nothing could possibly happen. And that he could never mistake it for anything more than a friendship.

✿

The first time Roberta took off her shirt in front of Lee, she was terrified. He asked her if she was sure she wanted to do it. She was, but was absolutely certain that the minute she did, the relationship would be over.

As Roberta unbuttoned her shirt, her hands were shaking. She was still in the middle of reconstruction, so her left breast had been pumped much larger than her right. It didn't even have a nipple. Lee just stared at Roberta's face.

"You don't think I'm going to care, do you? The rest of your body could be scarred up and down and I wouldn't care."

Lee kept his eyes on Roberta's face. Then he looked down. And back up at Roberta's face. "Is that it? Do you think I'm going to leave you now?"

Roberta started to cry.

"I'm never going to leave you," Lee said.

⋘∞⋙

In retrospect, Roberta decided that treatment wasn't actually the worst time to date. She didn't need Lee to take her to fancy restaurants or Broadway plays. She just wanted to sit in the park and talk.

And Lee's touch meant more than any man's had before her breast cancer.

"Can you feel my hand on your breast?" he asked.

"No," she said. "I cannot feel it physically, but emotionally, your touch is better than anything I can imagine."

Return to Normal Life

Roberta finished with her six cycles of chemotherapy. Now she could return to "normal life." But it was tough to figure out how to just be normal, how to stop thinking of herself as sick. During treatment, Roberta knew how to act. She was recuperating from surgery, surviving chemotherapy. Everything she had to do was laid out for her, from when to take her medicine and when to eat to how much sleep she needed. But now, treatment was over.

"See you in six months," the oncologist said.

"Six months?" Roberta responded. "You can't just send me away. What am I supposed to do now?" She wanted an extra dose of chemo for good luck. People had warned her that she was going to feel scared about losing her chemo team, that it would be a very emotional time. But she hadn't anticipated the extent of her anxiety.

Early on in the process, a friend and fellow survivor told Roberta, "You're not going to believe this, but breast cancer was the best thing that ever happened to me." At the time, she thought her friend was crazy. But now she absolutely agrees, "One hundred percent."

Six months after she finished treatment, Roberta made a number of changes in her life. Before, when people invited her to events, she would often say, "No, thank you, I'm too busy." But after breast cancer, she says, "I wouldn't miss it for the world." She spends as much time as she can with friends and family. She prefers to go out to dinner or sit on the couch and talk rather than watch movies or theater. "I am the person I want to be," she explains. "I wouldn't go back to the person I was before, wouldn't change this for anything in the world."

Much as she likes to anticipate and to manage, the most important question in Roberta's life—will the cancer come back?—is out of her hands. As she tells Lee, "We don't have a guarantee. We're going to be together as much as we can, as long as we can. We'll take it as it comes. And we'll go through it again if we have to."

So she tries to control, and balance, the rest of her life. She is cutting down her work schedule, starting by taking the weekends off. Roberta cares deeply about her consulting firm and her career. She feels grateful to her colleagues for their help, and to the work itself for taking her mind off breast cancer. And she is truly delighted to be able to return to the job with full energy.

"Don't work too hard," a friend said to her recently.

"I don't know about that," Roberta responded. "It feels great to work too hard. It really does. I want two things: I want to have time for my friends and family—and I want to work hard. There *is* life after breast cancer, and often it is a much better life."

Roberta and Lee have gotten married and moved to Houston. After having a prophylactic mastectomy of her remaining breast, Roberta has given birth to two little girls. She is director of cancer services at a large hospital, which is slightly less hectic than consulting. Roberta is one of the founders of the Young Survival Coalition, an international, nonprofit network of breast cancer survivors and supporters dedicated to the concerns and issues that are specific to young women with breast cancer. She devotes her spare time to promoting awareness of breast cancer among young women and has been honored for her efforts by the Susan G. Komen Breast Cancer Foundation. She is now in good health.

□ □ □

HOW DO I REGAIN CONTROL OF MY BODY?

*❧ Lanita, 31: Marathon Runner

AT TEN IN THE MORNING, an hour before the race was scheduled to begin, Lanita stretched out on the Staten Island side of the Verrazano-Narrows Bridge, one of the world's longest suspension bridges. Lanita was surrounded by roughly twenty-nine thousand other runners. Their ages ranged from adolescent to pushing a century, but most of the runners were, like Lanita, in their thirties. Everyone was eating, drinking, stretching, or waiting in line for the portable toilets. November's brisk seven-mile-per-hour wind made the forty-one-degree temperature feel even colder than Lanita had foreseen. But that was probably best; she'd warm up soon enough. She ran a hand through her straight blond hair. She was anxious to begin the 26.2-mile race, to accomplish the goal she had set for herself eleven months earlier in a lonely San Francisco hotel room. She was going to regain control over her body, prove to herself that breast cancer hadn't destroyed her.

Alone in a Hotel Room

It was just runner's nipple, Lanita told herself in May 1997, shortly after her thirty-first birthday. She was thinking about the scaling on her right breast that wasn't healing, the itchiness that just wouldn't go away. After all, she ran four to five miles a day and lifted weights two or three times a week. Plenty of opportunity for sweat to collect on her slim, five-foot, eight-inch body, plenty of opportunity for clothing to chafe. The sore was more of an annoyance than anything else, really. But she knew she ought to get it checked out, just in case.

Lanita had gotten so used to the sore that she didn't even remember exactly when it first appeared. It had already been there for three or four months by the time she went for her routine gynecologic appointment. The doctor agreed that it was probably runner's nipple and gave Lanita the name of a dermatologist to check it out. Lanita stuck the phone number in her wallet and promptly forgot about it.

She didn't think about the dermatologist again until it was time to set up her next biannual gynecology appointment the following January. The scaling hadn't healed and Lanita knew her doctor was going to ask what the dermatologist had said. So she hunted around her one-bedroom apartment on Manhattan's Upper East Side, found the name of the dermatologist, and made an appointment. The dermatologist, too, thought that the sore was runner's nipple. He prescribed an ointment for her to use for ten days.

A week and a half later, the sore still hadn't gone away. The dermatologist decided to perform a biopsy.

Meanwhile, Lanita continued with her job, fitting a new San Francisco facility with telecommunications and other electronic equipment. She flew to the West Coast for three-day trips every few weeks, working ten or more hours a day. The reward for her hectic work life was a Broadway or off-Broadway show followed by a candlelit meal on Restaurant Row with her husband, Tom.

On a Wednesday afternoon in January, Lanita sat alone in her Bay Area Park Hyatt room, checking her voicemail messages. A message from her gynecologist mentioned some confusion about the biopsy that the dermatologist had done, and she wanted to talk to Lanita about it. Lanita was puzzled. Why didn't the gynecologist just pick up the phone and call the dermatologist herself?

Feeling frustrated, Lanita phoned the dermatologist directly. His nurse said that he was with a patient and would call her back shortly. While she waited, Lanita wondered what was going on. Her gynecologist didn't usually leave cryptic messages after a routine exam. Finally, the hotel phone rang.

"First of all, I don't like to do this over the phone," the dermatologist began. "But under the circumstances, I feel the need to tell you that the test results came back. It's breast cancer. A type of breast cancer called Paget's disease. I recommend you come back to New York."

Lanita's fingers flew over the telephone buttons. She called Tom, her husband of seven and a half years, at work and told him. "The first thing to do is to get you home," he said. She phoned her dermatologist again, who said that he had made an appointment for her with a breast surgeon for further testing. Then she called her parents. Her mother knew about the sore that wouldn't heal, knew the doctor had taken a biopsy. "It's malignant," Lanita said. "And it's breast cancer."

Lanita raided the hotel room mini-bar, extracting both Scotch bottles and placing them on the nightstand. Then she sat on the carpeted floor between the two double beds and continued dialing, staring at the two little bottles of Scotch. She phoned the front desk to say that she would be checking out shortly, that there had been a medical emergency. She didn't mention that it was *her* medical emergency.

Finally, Lanita pushed the bottles aside and sat up straight. She decided, sitting on the floor of her hotel room, that she was not going to let this disease beat her. She was going to stick with her plan of running the New York City Marathon that coming November, just eleven months away. When she completed those 26.2 miles, she would know she had beaten breast cancer.

On the flight home, Lanita tried to rest. When the plane landed at JFK airport, she took a car service home. After holding her emotions in check for hours, Lanita opened the door to her apartment, saw her tall, clean-shaven husband, and burst into tears.

The Long Shadow of Cancer

Lanita thought about her three aunts who had been diagnosed with breast cancer and were still alive decades after their diagnoses. The closest, in terms of both bloodline and friendship, was Aunt Jan. All her life, Lanita had heard that she was like her Aunt Jan. She had Jan's straight blond hair, her fair skin, her delicate hands and feet, and her dry sense of humor. Now, it seemed, she had breast cancer like her as well. Aunt Jan had been diagnosed first at age thirty, then again thirteen years later. Despite the family history, Lanita was not prepared for her own terrifying diagnosis.

Tom made Lanita take a shower and put on her pajamas, even though it was now about seven o'clock in the morning in Manhattan and the apartment was bright with eastern sunlight. He turned down the bed and helped Lanita into it. Then he slipped off his penny loafers and crawled under the covers with her. The two of them held each other and waited for the gynecologist to call. The wait was uncomfortable, the room heavy with silence. Then the phone rang, echoing in the small space.

"There's one good thing in all of this," the gynecologist began. "Your breast cancer is not invasive, so it probably won't kill you. I mean, it might if you were to leave it alone, but not at this point. We caught it early enough."

Lanita thought about how the fear of breast cancer had always stalked her. When she was twenty-six years old and living in Minneapolis, she had asked her gynecologist to do a baseline mammogram. She wanted to be checked and to have a comparison for use as she got older. She told the gynecologist about her family history.

"I don't want to talk to you about that until you're thirty-five," the doctor had said. "Just put it out of your mind, it's not an issue. Mammograms aren't that accurate until you're at least thirty-five years old."

Lanita found another doctor, a woman, who was willing to do the baseline mammogram. And here she was, four years shy of her previous gynecologist's magic number, at age thirty-one, confronted with the diagnosis of breast cancer.

"Take Them Both"

The next day, Tom and Lanita went to meet the breast surgeon. The doctor told them that Paget's disease is a rare type of breast cancer that accounts for about 1 percent of all breast cancers. Then the surgeon enumerated the options: removal of the nipple only, removal of one breast, or removal of both breasts.

"Take them both, they're small," Lanita said, laughing.

"Don't say that," the breast surgeon responded. "Or I'll take you seriously."

"I *am* serious."

Lanita and Tom hadn't discussed this decision in advance. In fact, Lanita hadn't even really thought it through herself. In light of her family history, Lanita wanted both breasts removed preventively, a procedure called prophylactic double mastectomy. She never wanted to have this experience again, never wanted to hear a doctor tell her she had breast cancer again. She turned to look at Tom; he nodded.

"You are entitled to get a second opinion," the breast surgeon said.

"The only second opinion I want is a rereading of the pathology report," Lanita said. "I want someone else to verify it." (The second reading was positive as well.)

Four years before diagnosis, Lanita had set herself the goal of running a marathon. The first year, she ran a five-kilometer race; the second, she ran a 10K; the third, she ran a half-marathon; this year, she was slated to run a marathon, the New York City Marathon.

She'd run for years, doing about twenty miles a week wherever she went. She'd run in Barbados, she'd run in Trinidad. She'd found that it was a good way to see the sights a tourist might otherwise miss.

But Lanita didn't consider herself an athlete. An eleven-minute-miler who occasionally did a ten- or nine-and-a-half-minute mile, she ran through just two or three pairs of running shoes a year. In her opinion, a true athlete runs a six-minute mile and wears out three or four pairs of shoes a year. Just because she wasn't an athlete, though, didn't mean she wasn't serious about the sport.

Now, sitting in the doctor's office, Lanita had one more question for the breast surgeon.

"Can I run a marathon after all this?"

"I don't see why not," the doctor responded with a smile. "I don't see why you would want to, but I don't see why you couldn't."

Choosing Her Body's Future

Six days after she heard the diagnosis, Lanita met with her plastic surgeon. The plastic surgeon was part of a team of women doctors and specialists assembled by her breast surgeon. Lanita had long since decided to see only women gynecologists because she felt they were more apt to understand a woman's response to a yeast infection or a pregnancy than a man was. Lanita found she preferred other women specialists as well. "It's kind of cool when you tell your plastic surgeon that you don't want your reconstructed nipples to look like you're cold for the rest of your life—and she understands," she told her mother.

Lanita had no trouble deciding how to remove the cancer from her body, but the question of reconstruction was far more complicated. She didn't want implants; she didn't like the idea of having them replaced every fifteen years. She wanted this part of her life finished.

Lanita seriously considered a TRAM (transverse rectus abdominus muscle) flap procedure, which would involve moving muscle, fat, and tissue from her abdomen to her chest and molding them into a replacement breast.

As if deciding between a TRAM flap procedure and implants wasn't enough, Lanita was also faced with the question of children. Long ago, she had decided that she didn't want to have children until after she was thirty-five, partly to have time to establish her career and partly because she was never really certain she could get pregnant. In her early twenties, Lanita had had a bad case of pelvic inflammatory disease, which she was told often impairs fertility but has no known connection to cancer.

"I guess I need to decide if I ever want to have a child," Lanita said to Tom in a quiet voice.

"You are my first concern. We need to do whatever is best for you, physically and emotionally."

"If I want to have a child, I can't have a TRAM flap procedure, because a mesh-lined stomach can't carry a fetus to term." She paused. "But if I'm never going to get pregnant, I may as well have my tubes tied while I'm on the operating table." She turned to the surgeon. "When would be the best time to do that?"

"Probably while you're there on the operating table for the TRAM flap procedure," her surgeon replied.

That night, Lanita lay in bed and shuddered as she pictured herself on an operating table, surrounded by three or four doctors—her breast surgeon, her plastic surgeon, her gynecologist, and possibly an additional plastic surgeon—all wielding scalpels.

❦

Lanita collected information on breast cancer in general and Paget's disease and the TRAM flap procedure in particular. For technical questions, she approached a doctor friend; for psychological insights, she spoke with her aunts, especially Aunt Jan. She combed through bookstores. She read about the technical medical details and learned a slew of medical terms—invasive versus noninvasive cancers, positive nodes versus negative nodes, saline versus silicone implants—and the ramifications of each. After a while, Lanita found she couldn't handle any more information. She put the books and notes away, deciding that they couldn't make the decisions. She had to. She went with her gut and opted for saline implants instead of the TRAM flap. Once she decided, she felt calm.

Lanita took her pending breast reconstruction as an opportunity to design the figure she'd always wanted. And what she wanted was small. She had danced when she was younger and had always envied the dancer's body shape. Many women tell their plastic surgeons that they want their reconstructed breasts to be the same size as or larger than the originals. But Lanita ordered the smallest size of implants available.

Boot Camp for Breast Surgery

The day after they'd scheduled the surgery, Tom announced, "Boot camp starts today. We're going to get you in the best shape possible."

Lanita knew that not everybody trained for surgery, but she figured the more muscles she built up in advance, the easier it would be to regain her strength later. From that day on, Lanita ran daily, bench-pressed at the gym every day, and tightened her chest muscles as much as possible. Tom rousted her out of bed every morning at 6:30, then rolled over and went back to sleep.

Lanita went back to her job a week after receiving her diagnosis. She gradually told her colleagues, her staff, and the office manager about her diagnosis. Everyone was very supportive. Her company agreed to allow her to take as long as she needed to recuperate, without having her pay docked.

At the Hospital

On the day of the surgery, no one noticed the brisk March weather. The family waited in the hospital during the six-hour procedure: double mastectomy and reconstruction.

"We examined her breast completely and didn't find any spreading," the breast surgeon announced as she came out of the operating room. "It was contained at the nipple level. Her other breast checked out fine."

As she lay in the hospital bed, Lanita wondered if she would ever put her running shoes on again. But when she took her first tentative steps three days after surgery, holding tightly on to her mother, she was elated. "These are my first steps toward the marathon finishing line," she said. Just six months to go.

While Lanita recuperated in the hospital, Tom visited every day. Visiting hours started at 11:00 AM, but he broke the rules and stopped by before work. He wasn't the only visitor; Lanita's family and friends came by regularly.

The day after surgery, a Reach for Recovery volunteer came to her room. Dressed in a little white skirt, she explained, "I just finished playing three sets of tennis."

To Lanita, the volunteer looked old—probably ten, fifteen years older than she—and Lanita had a hard time accepting her message.

"I just want you to know that it's not always going to be this way," the volunteer offered.

"Go away," Lanita replied.

Four days after surgery, Lanita's plastic surgeon signed the paperwork to check her out of the hospital. Lanita's breast surgeon also came by. "You look fine," she said. "Go home."

The hospital wouldn't permit Lanita to leave except in a wheelchair, but one couldn't be found. Lanita sat in the lobby, demanding, "Get me a wheelchair or I'm walking out of here."

The orderly finally located a wheelchair, but it didn't have footrests.

"I'm fine! I'll hold my feet up," said an impatient Lanita. "I'm going *now*." As the orderly pushed her down the hall, Lanita held her legs straight out from her hips until they got to the car.

A Normal Life within Reach

Lanita might have been able to leave the hospital, but she was far from self-sufficient. Her entire chest was wrapped in bandages and she could barely lift either arm above her waist. The first thing she wanted to do when she got home was to take a bath to wash the smell and feel of the hospital off her body. So Tom washed her hair over the sink, thinking that would be easier than in the bath. Then he gently took off her clothing, ran the bath water, and helped her into the tub. When she was comfortably settled, he scrubbed her arms and legs with a washcloth and soap, gently washed her face. He helped her out of the tub and toweled her dry, then helped her step into her sweatpants. Finally, he gently pulled a T-shirt over her head and down over her bandages. He helped her bathe every day for weeks.

Lanita spent the latter half of March and early April recuperating at home. She rested and walked around the neighborhood. She went to stretching classes and read romance novels, which line a wall of her living room in floor-to-ceiling bookshelves. Each week, she went to her plastic surgeon's office to have more saline pumped into her breast implants to stretch out the muscles.

Survivor Suggestions on Interacting with Doctors and Other Health Care Providers

☐ *Get a second opinion*. It is your right, you're worth it, *and it could save your life*.

☐ If someone mentions the possibility of breast cancer, even if they think you're too young for the disease, follow up.

☐ Interview doctors until you find one you feel comfortable with, who shares your feelings about diagnosis and treatment, and who is convenient for your lifestyle.

☐ Try to find a doctor who is able to think about your whole body.

☐ If your doctor makes you uncomfortable, either medically or emotionally, consider switching. It is *your* choice.

☐ Be an informed patient: Write down all information in a notebook; bring a list of questions to each appointment; read all reports; look at all films. Many women recommend bringing a friend or relative to each appointment to help you remember and sort through all the information.

☐ Make informed decisions about your doctors and treatment plan.

☐ Push your doctor or health insurance company or HMO to get the care you need.

☐ Ask your doctor about any symptoms you may experience; there may be a simple solution and there is no reason to suffer needlessly.

☐ Remember the possibility of human fallibility among medical professionals; question your doctors.

☐ Consider prophylactic surgery, a very personal choice.

Lanita's mother stayed with the couple during the first week after surgery. When she left New York and Tom returned to work, Lanita was alone. Tom wasn't sure how to take care of Lanita. Should he cater to her every need? Or should he set small goals for her, to help her get back to normal? He took a cue from her marathoner's step-by-step technique and decided on a tough-love approach.

The first day Lanita was home by herself, Tom asked her what she wanted to eat for lunch and left it out on the counter for her. The second day, he just left.

"Aren't you going to get anything for me?" Lanita asked.

"Get a chair and get it yourself."

"You're such a stoic German," Lanita teased him. She knew that the only way she was going to get better was to push herself a little harder every day. But that didn't mean she wanted to.

Her first goal was a cup of coffee. The mugs and sugar bowl were in the shoulder-high cabinets. She lifted her arm, but it didn't quite make it that high. She felt like there were rubber bands running down her arm, keeping her from moving freely. She lifted her arm again. After several tries, she pulled down a cream-colored mug. She filled the mug with coffee and set it on the counter. Next she stretched up for the sugar bowl, reaching it on her fourth try. At last she sat down at her kitchen table. She'd had cups of coffee that were hotter, but never one she'd worked harder for.

Her goal for the next day: reach the plates on the shelf *above* the mugs.

A week or two after her surgery, Lanita had heard some other breast cancer patients mentioning an exercise called "walking the walls." Most women are told to do this exercise daily after a mastectomy to regain mobility. The action involves holding the arm straight out until the fingers reach a wall, then "walking" the fingers up the wall, higher and higher each day.

"Should I be walking the wall?" Lanita asked her breast surgeon.

"We're not worried about you," the doctor replied. "We know you're going to figure out a way to do it on your own. Your daily living is going to get you back into shape."

Lanita had met some other young breast cancer survivors she liked and formed an informal support group. "When we get together, we start talking about how when we're sixty years old and all of our friends have breasts that sag down to their knees, we'll still have perky ones!"

Relearning to Run

When Lanita returned to work in April, she also got her doctor's approval to begin running again. Tom was terrified. He hated to run, but he went with her to Central Park at East 90th Street and they ran together. It was more of a spirited walk than anything else. But with each step, Lanita tried to relearn to trust her body the way she had before the cancer. Each footfall was a step away from cancer and toward crossing the Verrazano-Narrows Bridge in November. She knew that if she could run all 26 miles and 385 yards of the New York City Marathon, then breast cancer hadn't beaten her.

By now, breast cancer didn't control Lanita's life; running did. Four days a week she ran, starting with shorter runs and working her way up to fifteen to twenty miles a week. Eventually, Tom took up golfing to entertain himself during Lanita's long absences. She didn't just run; she also lifted weights two or three times a week and swam regularly.

"Marathoners aren't normal people," Lanita explained to her doctor. "If you were normal, you wouldn't choose it. It's a huge physical undertaking, but it's also mental. About 80 percent mental." For Lanita, the goal wasn't recuperating from cancer. The goal was running the marathon.

Cancer slowed her down. Cancer made her train differently. Cancer even knocked her feet out from under her. But she couldn't dwell on the cancer. Lanita focused every single bit of her energy on the marathon. It made her do things she might not have done if she weren't so focused on exercise.

To train for the marathon, Lanita did two eighteen-mile runs and a twenty-mile run. Two of these were in Central Park, while Tom played golf, and the third run she did while in Dallas visiting her parents. Her parents made her carry her cell phone and met her at the nine-mile mark with fruit and Gatorade. "Are you sure you don't want to run the Race for the Cure?" they asked.

"Maybe next year," said Lanita. "But I set my sights on the New York City Marathon before I was diagnosed, and that's what I'm going to do."

Making Her Mark

To mark the end of her battle with breast cancer, Lanita went downtown to a tattoo parlor in the Flatiron District, just north of Greenwich Village. She wanted a pink ribbon planted on her right breast, the one where the cancer had been. The tattooist, Dragon Fly, had a shaved head, tattoos on her arms and neck, and a pierced lower lip.

"Why do you want a tattoo?" Dragon Fly asked, staring at the conservatively dressed young businesswoman who looked so different from her other clients.

"It marks that I am finished with breast cancer," Lanita told her. "Like the period at the end of a sentence."

26.2

Lanita ran the New York City Marathon eleven months after she was diagnosed with breast cancer and nine months after surgery. Her parents and mother-in-law came to watch, as did her three sisters-in-law. Her family and friends met her at the eighteen-mile mark with orange slices, Kleenex, and a calculator to check her time.

As Lanita crossed into Marcus Garvey Park in Harlem and began to see Central Park up ahead, she knew she would meet her goal and finish the race. The last four hundred yards were steep, but she had already met her uphill challenge. Each step put breast cancer further behind her. At mile twenty-five, she saw Tom and her parents waving. At that moment, Lanita knew that she had stared down breast cancer. And the cancer had blinked first. With a last burst of energy, she crossed the finish line, puffing her way under the white banner. Elated, thrilled beyond her expectations, and exhausted, Lanita collected her Finisher's Medal, blanket, water, snack bag, and long-stemmed red rose.

Lanita finished the marathon in five hours and forty-four minutes, averaging a thirteen-minute mile. Not amazing. But her goal was never speed, it was completion. "Even before I began this marathon," Lanita says, "I had already run the race of my life. And I won."

Shortly after she finished treatment, Lanita and Tom made plans to adopt a child from Eastern Europe. Tom was killed in a plane crash before they were able to complete those plans. Six months after the crash, Lanita adopted a little girl, whom she named Elliott, on her own. She now lives in Kansas City with her new husband. Lanita is another of the co-founders, along with Roberta, of the Young Survival Coalition, an international support, activist, and outreach group geared to young women with breast cancer. Lanita remains in good health.

      □ □ □

Regaining control is a theme that runs throughout the stories in this book. From the moment a woman hears the diagnosis of breast cancer, she must try to put back together the pieces of her life. The feeling of loss of control—and the subsequent need to regain it—affects every woman differently. Some women stick with skills and interests that they were invested in before diagnosis; others take the opportunity to change priorities or goals.

Both Roberta and Lanita regained control over their lives and their bodies by determining exactly what they could control and what they could not. They could choose the course of treatment, but couldn't guarantee it would work. So they educated themselves as much as possible, then let their hearts lead them to the right decisions.

Roberta, the consummate manager, brought her organizational and people skills to the task of regaining control, as did Anne, whom you'll meet in the next chapter. Lanita used her personal strength and determination to break each major goal down into manageable little steps and meet every challenge head-on. Mary and Sarah chose to focus their energies inward, whereas Nora didn't feel in control until she returned to her career.

Every woman is an individual, every body and its diagnosis is distinct, yet strength, determination, and an ability to focus on personal assets are universally critical to regaining control over life and body.

Survivor Suggestions on Regaining Control

☐ Having breast cancer is not within your control, but how you treat it is. Take control of treatment by doing medical research and by thinking about your own needs and desires.

☐ Remember: Your life is what you make of it. Use your breast cancer diagnosis as an opportunity to change your life, to make it what you want it to be.

☐ Sometimes setting a goal and sticking with it can help pull you through treatment. Decide what you want out of life and figure out how to make it happen. This may mean periodically setting new goals for yourself.

☐ Realize that your priorities may change as a result of having a life-threatening disease.

☐ Cancer may force you do to some things differently, but it doesn't necessarily force you to stop altogether.

☐ Play to your strengths: Use your organizational skills, determination, and other personal assets to help you handle breast cancer and life after.

☐ Do your own research; don't just rely on what doctors tell you. Learn enough to feel comfortable with your decisions.

☐ Continue to exercise during treatment, within the limits of what your body can stand.

☐ When family and friends offer to help, take them up on the offer. Figure out what each person in your life can do to help; some are better at running errands than at attending chemotherapy sessions. And don't be afraid to ask for help.

Chapter Two

Work and Career

When Anne told her supervisor that she had breast cancer,
he said, "Oh, I'm sorry, but will you still be able to
join us for a conference call tomorrow?"

A WOMAN'S CAREER IS AN IMPORTANT PART of her identity, and women in their twenties and thirties are often at critical stages of career development. The choice of job and its subsequent path influences a woman's interests, her circle of friends, and the structure of her day-to-day life. It affects how a woman views herself and how "successful" she feels.

Being diagnosed with breast cancer changes all of that. It forces women to assess their careers and consider whether they have made active choices or if they've been just drifting, waiting, or making do. A breast cancer diagnosis shines a spotlight on the fragility of life, which often prompts soul-searching. And treatment often causes a slowing down or a break in activity, which gives a woman time for intense thought. As a result, women's careers rarely continue to glide along in the status quo after treatment.

Helen's career was shaken up by her disease. Before diagnosis, she was a high-powered litigator. But when breast cancer disrupted her life, she decided to change careers and became an advocate for social change, which she feels brings greater meaning to her life. By contrast, breast cancer helped Anne realize how fulfilling her chosen career is for her; after diagnosis, she went back to school and earned an Ivy League MBA, then took her business acumen to Wall Street.

Other women may decide to continue along the same career path but change their priorities. Janis, for instance, chose to spend less time in the office and place greater emphasis on her personal life. She now limits her work hours "to only forty or fifty hours a week."

Health insurance is another important work-related issue. Prior to diagnosis, Nora had worked as a freelancer in film art direction, which meant she had no health insurance. As a result, when she was diagnosed, she had to quit working and go on welfare just to qualify for Medicaid, which paid for her health care. The boredom of unemployment, along with fears for her future employment, contributed to her depression during treatment. Without her identity as a worker, she had to redefine herself. Ultimately, she went back to her film career with even greater enthusiasm.

Breast cancer can prompt a change in career or urge a realignment of professional priorities. Or it can give a woman a place to focus her energy and thoughts or lend a feeling of normalcy during a very stressful period. The stories in this chapter reflect a range of experiences.

WHAT IF MY CAREER IS NO LONGER FULFILLING?

🐉 Helen,* 32: The Career Switch

HELEN WORKED AT ONE OF THE BEST-KNOWN LAW FIRMS in New England and had a large, swanky office overlooking the Boston harbor. The firm provided gourmet lunches and dinners made by its own

*Not her real name

chef, and Helen earned a six-figure salary and got to "play with the big boys." As a senior associate, she had carved out a niche for herself doing intellectual property litigation and was in line to make partner. She enjoyed the competitive side to litigation and loved keeping up with the latest technological developments and meeting cutting-edge innovators.

Helen wasn't thrilled with the eighty- to hundred-hour workweeks; she would rather have spent more time with her family, friends, and husband, Dennis. But it certainly had its rewards. She and Dennis enjoyed a five-bedroom colonial in a tony Boston suburb, exotic beach vacations, and dining at Boston's finest restaurants.

Then, at age thirty-two, Helen was diagnosed with breast cancer.

Heading for the Bar

Helen hadn't sought out a high-powered, highly competitive life. When she got her law degree, she simultaneously earned a master's degree in public administration (MPA), a management degree for working in nonprofits and government. She planned to work for a nonprofit organization or do legal services work. But she really shone at Syracuse Law. She was in the top 10 percent of her class, served on the law review, and was an all-around stellar student. The Socratic method scared her, but it unearthed her competitive instincts and showed her a new side of herself, a side that thrived on what she described as the "chest-thumping, testosterone-ridden" style of oral advocacy. And she was bored in the undemanding MPA program, which made law seem even more exciting by comparison.

When she spoke with a career counselor at the university to plan her internship between the second and third years of grad school, the counselor was surprised. "With your grades, you could work at one of the top firms in Boston. Why do you want to go into legal services?"

"I want to spend my life helping people," Helen explained.

"Well, you have a lot of school debt. If you want to have ten room-mates and be on a tight budget while you pay back your student loans, you can work at legal services. But if you want the best training, the best pedigree, and the ability to write your own ticket, you should explore working at a large corporate firm."

The argument was compelling. And that, Helen remembers, was the end of her idealistic dream.

⚜

The career counselor was right. With her credentials, it wasn't difficult for Helen to land a summer internship at one of the fastest-growing law firms in New England. The firm focused on high tech and venture capital, two particularly vibrant sectors in the early 1990s. It was Helen's first time in such a corporate environment and she loved it. She decided to go back after graduation.

The third year of law school was a cakewalk because Helen already had a job lined up. She didn't have to pound the pavement; she knew how much she could spend on an apartment and still pay off her student loans—everything was set. All she had to worry about was her course work and preparing for the bar examination, which she passed easily.

At the Top of Her Game

Helen loved being a corporate litigator and worked on a variety of cases at the firm. A huge patent-infringement case piqued her interest in intellectual property. She enjoyed acting as conduit between the technical people and the judge, translating intellectual property ideas into lay terms. She was thrilled—and vindicated—that the law firm corridors were lined with Ivy League degrees. It had always been a bone of contention for her that hadn't been accepted at any of the best schools.

Now she was at the top of her game and constantly receiving positive feedback on her work. But exciting as it was, she began to have reservations about the number of hours she was putting in. A short day for Helen began at nine in the morning and lasted until seven o'clock at night. When she had serious deadlines, she often went into the office before six and stayed until eight or nine at night. It was both a blessing and a curse that she could work those hours, that she had no family or other obligations pulling her out the front door once the sun set. Everyone at the firm wanted the associates to be available, but they ignored the pattern: Associates tended to peter out after a few years of those work hours.

In her fourth year of practice, Helen met Dennis. "It's a good thing I got to know you," she told him after they'd been dating for a while. "I was starting to worry that I wasn't going to find anyone, that I was going to become the cat lady of Cambridge." Dennis had an MBA and worked in high-tech ventures, usually with start-ups. "I'm glad you work in business, because I wanted to avoid lawyers," she said. Dating was a challenge for the two of them and required synchronizing Palm Pilots and coordinating frequent-flier miles. But they managed to sneak in more than a few romantic dinners and a couple of trips to the theater. After three years of dating, they were married in a small private ceremony at a historic Boston mansion.

Not long after they got married, Helen and Dennis began to think about starting a family. Helen went off the pill and they tried casually to get pregnant for about six months, though without any luck. They chalked their failure up to Dennis's hectic travel schedule and Helen's crazy work hours.

Then Helen's breasts began to hurt—both of them. The pain was so great that she could hardly bring herself to put on a shirt. She couldn't connect the pain to any particular point in her cycle, and she made an appointment to see her gynecologist, who was on maternity leave at the time. Helen ended up seeing a new doctor who had just completed her residency program. Helen was concerned; she generally preferred older, more experienced doctors.

"I don't feel anything on the manual exam," said the doctor.

"It hurts less than usual today," Helen said. "It's like getting a haircut; your hair looks great on the day you're getting it cut."

The doctor laughed. "Maybe I'm crazy," she added, "but let's just send you for a mammogram to make sure there's nothing there. I'm probably violating all of the guidelines because you're under forty and don't have any family history of breast cancer. But let's check it out just to be sure." She played down the possibility of breast cancer, explaining that Helen was probably experiencing cyclical pain related to ovulation.

Helen agreed with the doctor; the test was probably unnecessary. But she went for the appointment.

Serious Business

"There are microcalcifications in your left breast," said the radiologist.

"Could you repeat that word?" asked Helen. She'd never heard the term before and was going to have to look it up; she realized it would soon become very important in her life.

"Microcalcification," repeated the radiologist. "It looks highly suspicious for a malignancy. I suggest you get yourself to a breast surgeon soon to have a biopsy."

"A biopsy?" Helen was stunned; she was sure her gynecologist had been overly cautious in ordering the mammogram. But a biopsy meant serious business.

"I recommend you have an excisional biopsy, not just a needle biopsy, because with calcifications they could end up testing some tissue that's not malignant and missing some that is."

Several weeks elapsed between the mammogram and the biopsy. By now, several doctors had told Helen that they would be surprised if the results came back benign. She began to prepare herself for a diagnosis of breast cancer. Helen later said that waiting for the definitive diagnosis was one of the hardest parts of the whole experience. She learned, incidentally, that the breast pain was unrelated to the cancer and was connected with her ovulation cycle, as her gynecologist had suspected.

Helen and Dennis also used this time between diagnostic tests to do research. "That's our way of coping," Dennis said.

"Knowledge is power," Helen agreed.

"We have time to investigate options," Helen said. "Breast cancer is rarely a medical emergency." They knew that the standard treatment for breast cancer was surgery, chemotherapy, and radiation, and they went to breast surgeon and oncologist appointments together, armed with a list of questions and a tape recorder. They were particularly thorough in interviewing oncologists because Helen figured that this was the person she would see most during treatment and after. She thought it was important that she like the person who would give her chemotherapy.

Helen told her managing partner and other people in the office what was going on. Her goal was to finish the project she was working on because she knew if the test came back positive she would take a leave of absence. She didn't see how she could keep working such long hours during treatment, so she would go on short-term disability.

Ten days after the biopsy, the doctor called Helen with the results. It was, indeed, breast cancer. Helen had been prepared for the diagnosis, but that didn't make it any easier. In her head, she kept seeing a marquee with lights going around that said "*death... death... death.*"

Helen called her managing partner and told him she had been definitively diagnosed and was going to take a leave of absence. The partner was supportive of her decision and told her to take it easy. "We'll see you when you're done with treatment," he said.

That night, Helen told Dennis, "I've been looking for a mission, a philanthropic activity. I've been really involved in the Multiple Sclerosis Society because my father has the disease, but it just hasn't been my passion. But I think breast cancer is it. I think this is where I'm going to hang my hat."

The couple agreed to treat the cancer as aggressively as possible and figure out how to have children later. Interestingly, Helen continued to menstruate throughout chemotherapy and later. This is unusual—her nurse practitioner jokingly called her "Iron Ovaries."

※

Helen made it a point to bring a box of chocolates to her new gynecologist to express her gratitude. The lump was less than one centimeter in diameter, but it was growing aggressively. Because Helen was thirty-two, doctors probably wouldn't have done a baseline mammogram for another eight years; by then, her gynecologist suggested, the lump would likely have been palpable. But even if the cancer had been found just a few years later, Helen's prognosis would have been radically different; her cancer could well have been metastatic by that point.

"Every doctor lives to be able to do this for someone," her gynecologist said. "I'm so sorry for the diagnosis, but it was a lucky break that we found the cancer so early." Helen couldn't agree more.

"Now I'm going to send anybody for any test I want," the gynecologist added. "After this, I am totally justified."

❧

The first lumpectomy did not leave clean margins, so Helen had a second lumpectomy and a sentinel node biopsy. The sentinel node biopsy came back fine; the cancer had not spread to her lymph nodes, but the margins of her tumor still were not clean. "There is still a bit of DCIS [ductal carcinoma in situ] or atypical hyperplasia in your breast," said the doctor. "Radiation will probably get it all."

But Helen was nervous. "Do another lumpectomy," she said. "I'd rather be certain."

They agreed that Helen would begin chemotherapy and that the third lumpectomy would follow.

Helen was terrified of chemotherapy, having seen too many movies where people on chemo spent their days vomiting. But she took anti-nausea medication and never threw up. She was very tired, though. She tried to exercise throughout chemo, but in the last few months of treatment, even walking up a flight of stairs wore her out.

A New Project

Helen often coped with difficult situations by throwing herself into a new project wholeheartedly. Breast cancer was no exception. She sought out an organized group of young survivors in their twenties and thirties. She had been impressed with an organization in New

York City, but couldn't find a similar support group in Boston, so she helped form a Boston-area chapter of the New York organization, holding the first meeting in her new living room. She and Dennis had just moved in and had no furniture, so the fifteen participants perched on metal folding chairs. Helen found it empowering to see so many young women in the same situation as she. Helen continues to be involved with this group, and has also started the first Boston-area support group (unconnected to the New York group) for women forty and under with breast cancer. The group meets every two weeks, and there are typically ten to twelve participants every time.

Having a support group tremendously helped Helen deal with her breast cancer. Some women she met through the support group and elsewhere managed to stay positive throughout the whole experience. But Helen had lots of ups and downs. There were days when thinking about having a child filled her with joyful hope and days when it reminded her of the possibility of recurrence.

"Some women say it's a gift to be diagnosed with breast cancer because it creates insights," Helen told Dennis. "I would gladly be ignorant and vacuous," Helen smiled. "But I figured that if I took the time to assimilate the experience into my life and think about things I could do that will have a positive impact going forward, it could be a phenomenal learning tool and a phenomenal way to get to a place that a lot of people don't get to until they're much older, if at all. I always tell women who are newly diagnosed that life actually can get better from this," Helen said. "When you're first diagnosed, you think your life is ending, if not literally, then figuratively. Life as you know it is going to change."

"But doesn't it get better day by day?" Dennis asked.

"No, it's not a linear progression. At least for me, it's more like losing weight: I go up and down," Helen said slowly. "I can be terrified, sad, and elated all within the span of thirty minutes."

True Friends

Helen made many new friends through support groups and her advocacy work. She strengthened existing friendships and developed acquaintances into friends. Every day the mail carrier brought cards, and she received so many flowers she joked about opening up her own floral shop. People brought homemade macaroni and cheese, vegetarian lasagna, and other dishes she and Dennis could just reheat after a long day. It seemed as though just about everyone Helen had ever known took this opportunity to help out. Her friends reached out to her, inviting her to get together with them. They offered whatever she wanted: "If you want to go out, we'll go out. If you want us to come over and all just hang out in our pajamas, we can do that."

Having all these friends step up to the plate helped Helen realize the importance of not always trying to be self-sufficient. It was difficult for her to sit at the kitchen table while a friend washed the dinner dishes; she had to learn to let someone else unload her dishwasher and fold her laundry. Helen had always been able to give to her friends, but it took breast cancer for her to learn to receive.

Several close friends disappointed her. After learning that Helen had cancer, they rarely called and never offered to visit, even though they lived close by. Some of them made surprisingly insensitive remarks about breasts and breast cancer. Given the immensity of breast cancer, Helen has had a hard time letting bygones be bygones and has let some friendships fall by the wayside.

❧

After Helen finished treatment, she went for a fertility workup. It turned out that her egg reserves were somewhat lower than they had been before treatment, but she was still fertile.

Helen and Dennis were in a quandary. They didn't want to wait until Helen finished with tamoxifen, at age thirty-eight, to try to get pregnant. Her fertility would drop because of her age and they simply wanted to start having a family before then. But pregnancy could dramatically increase the chance that the cancer would come back.

Ultimately, they decided to adopt a daughter from China. "At the end of all this, we know we're going to end up with a child," said Dennis. "It's a long process, but it's predictable."

One Door Closes, Another Opens

After three surgeries, four months of chemotherapy, and another six weeks of radiation, it was a relief to be finished with treatment. But it wasn't the cause for celebration that Helen had initially envisioned. Helen and Dennis thought about throwing a party to celebrate the end of debilitating fatigue and hair thinning, but Helen ultimately vetoed it. "I'm really tired, I'm bald, I feel burned, and it's the middle of June. I've lost half my summer and I don't really feel psyched to celebrate." Instead, they spent a quiet weekend in New York.

Coming to the end of treatment also meant that Helen would have to make a final decision about her career. She found that her attitude toward work had changed. She couldn't imagine going back to work as a corporate litigator after this meaningful and life-altering experience. She believes that chemotherapy changes a person at the cellular level—not just at the hair follicles, but in the brain as well.

"After what I've been through, I just can't imagine going back to that chest-thumping world," Helen told Dennis.

"You help people by making sure your clients don't get robbed by big corporations trying to take advantage of their ideas," he replied. "And your clients have generally been pleased with your work."

"Yes, but it's just about moving money from one pocket to another. The problems I was helping them solve were about money and power, not personal and emotional issues. Intellectual property law doesn't have a huge impact on someone's life, like helping someone who's been diagnosed with breast cancer."

"So follow your heart," Dennis told her. And she did.

A Merger of Talents

Cutting back on practicing law freed up Helen's time to become involved with several breast cancer organizations. She joined the board of directors of the Massachusetts Breast Cancer Coalition, which emphasizes primary prevention of breast cancer. She gave talks for Check It Out, a program that brings breast cancer survivors to high schools to teach students about the disease.

Perhaps most important, Helen became regional coordinator for the Massachusetts and Rhode Island chapters of the Young Survival Coalition, founded by several women, including Roberta and Lanita from Chapter One. She devotes about twenty hours a week to the YSC.

Helen found that advocacy merged her myriad talents. It wedded the business experience, analytical skills, and "pushiness" she gained through legal work with the management and development training of her MPA and her strong interest in personal and emotional issues.

She continued to practice law part-time, mostly for the income. But it had become important to Helen that her work be socially relevant and meaningful. Her legal work involved a health care venture aimed at low-income seniors, which she found more satisfying than intellectual property litigation.

Helen enjoyed turning something very negative into something positive. She found it rewarding to help women, especially women newly diagnosed with breast cancer, who were at a very vulnerable place. She learned that the simplest things can do the greatest good: Just telling a newly diagnosed woman that there is someone of the same age with a similar diagnosis, just connecting women in their twenties and thirties up with other young breast cancer survivors, can create an incredible sense of relief. The group she started continued to meet once a month and eventually gained more than 150 members. Helen wanted to create an outlet for women, a way to create meaning out of their breast cancer experience.

Helen now says, "I just can't imagine my life without doing this advocacy work. The two worlds are so different: The world of the litigator is analytic and unemotional; you greet people with a handshake. In the breast cancer world, there is a lot of hugging, a lot of emotional availability. Women who have had breast cancer don't beat around the bush. They don't want to waste time on bullshit, and to be a litigator is to specialize in bullshit. I could deal with it before breast cancer and brush it off when it got annoying. But after breast cancer, my bullshit meter was on 'red alert.'"

Breast cancer has helped Helen find meaningful new work, and her new work has helped her find meaning in breast cancer. "Whether I die in five months or fifty years, I want to go out with the assurance that I made a difference in the world."

Helen now devotes most of her time to breast cancer advocacy. She and her husband are currently pursuing adopting a daughter from China. She is in good health.

       □ □ □

In a sense, Helen's story addresses two themes: changing careers and increasing social activism. And in both of these arenas, she has plenty of company. Many women switch careers as a result of their experience with breast cancer. Often, additional education is a part of this change. Not everyone is as fortunate as Helen to have already completed the necessary schooling. Barbara, for instance, went back for her associate's degree, which allowed her to move off the factory assembly line and into medical office work. Dawn attended nursing school and is now a labor and delivery nurse. Similarly, Jacquie changed course from an MBA to a doctoral program and now works in university administration.

Often, women who have had breast cancer find that they have a greater interest in social activism, particularly in areas related to breast cancer research funding or advocacy. Some start their own organizations. Roberta and Lanita were two of the founders of the Young Survival Coalition, Helen helped found the Massachusetts/ Rhode Island chapter of YSC, Mary started Rocky Mountain Team Survivor, and Janis is a founding member of the Silent Spring Institute, which researches environmental links to breast cancer.

Others work for existing organizations in various capacities. Paulette is very involved with the Susan G. Komen Foundation's Race for the Cure and now runs in the race with her daughter alongside her. Janis is active in fund-raising for the Massachusetts Breast Cancer

Coalition. Dana has used her work on college campuses to informally teach students about the disease. Barbara accompanied her doctor to Washington, D.C., to lobby her congressman against banning breast implants. Using her own situation as an example, Barbara made the case for keeping breast implants available, and safe, for all women—particularly those who had undergone mastectomies. And just about every survivor informally counsels other young women with the disease, particularly those who have been recently diagnosed. After experiencing breast cancer, many women do whatever they can to help others cope with the disease and work toward its elimination.

WHAT IF MY CAREER PRIORITIES CHANGE?

❧ Janis, 33: Setting Limits

JANIS BROUGHT *SWAN LAKE, GISELLE,* and the December perennial, *Nutcracker Suite,* to Boston. As theater manager for the Wang Center for the Performing Arts, the city's premier dance stage and home to the Boston Ballet, thirty-three-year-old Janis booked the productions, worked with show management, set ticket prices, and settled accounts with the shows. To do that, Janis put work before family; before friends; before Chris, her partner of ten years; and before her health.

An athletic woman with straight, salt-and-pepper hair, Janis lived in a condominium in Boston's South End. Originally from New York, she'd been in New England for more than a decade. She kept in close touch with her parents, now retired in Florida, and with her brother, Howard, who lived just a few blocks away.

Saying It Out Loud

The following April, Janis was doing her monthly breast exam in her morning shower and felt something in her left breast. "It can't be a lump," she said out loud. "I'll just wait a month for my period to cycle through." Then, as the shampoo ran down her short black hair and down her back, she changed her mind.

The test was inconclusive. The gynecologist referred Janis to a surgeon for a biopsy. An outpatient procedure, the biopsy was scheduled for just before Memorial Day, when Janis and Chris were planning to go to Cape Cod. Janis was a little nervous after the procedure, but decided to focus on enjoying her long weekend at the beach.

Because everything closed down for Memorial Day weekend, Janis didn't get the results of the biopsy for almost a week. She was sitting at her desk, rummaging through a morass of memos, when the telephone rang.

"Hi, Janis. This is your surgeon calling. We got the results of the biopsy."

"Oh." Janis tensed, unnerved at getting a call from her doctor at work and surprised to be getting the results of such a major test by telephone rather than in person.

"I'm sorry to have to tell you this, but it's breast cancer."

They set up an appointment, then Janis quickly got off the phone, her mind a blur. She sat back and let the diagnosis filter through her brain. She felt stunned more than anything. She decided that the only way to make the diagnosis seem *real* was to say it out loud, to tell people. Sitting at her desk, pen in her hand, she called Chris.

"Chris," she said. "I have breast cancer."

Without missing a beat, Chris said, "Okay...we're going to fight this together. We're going to gear up, we're going to march forward, and we're going to beat this." Janis could hear the tears in Chris's voice and was grateful for her partner's efforts to be upbeat.

Janis phoned her parents in Florida and listened to her mother sob into the telephone. "It's not so bad, Mom," Janis said, trying to provide her mother some comfort. "The doctor said we found it early, so I have a good chance of beating it." Her mother continued to cry. Finally, her father picked up the receiver and said, "Janis, I think we ought to go now. We'll call you back when your mother's feeling a little better, when we can be more helpful to you."

When Janis told her supervisor at work, her supervisor suggested she take the rest of the day off. "I'll have my mother give you a call. She had breast cancer, too, and maybe she has some suggestions."

Janis nodded gratefully. She could tell that she was going to need all the help she could get.

꿍

The next day, Janis decided that she didn't know enough about breast cancer. She needed an education in the disease. She hadn't known anyone with breast cancer before and there were so many terms to learn, so many tests and treatments to understand. She hit the bookstores and decided to talk to doctors, nurses, and breast cancer survivors.

Through her doctor, Janis met a woman who had received the same diagnosis ten years earlier, a woman who became her mentor. The woman had not only had a similar experience with breast cancer at a young age, but was also a therapist; they began to speak on the phone every few weeks. Her mentor always knew when to provide comfort, when to provide information, and when to tell Janis to buck up. They remain friends to this day.

After the lumpectomy, the breast surgeon scheduled a dissection of Janis's lymph nodes to determine whether any were cancerous. Chris attended the procedure, taking copious notes in the red spiral notebook they had purchased to track Janis's progress and treatment. "*Ths tst is good indicat. whether canc. has spread outside brst,*" Chris scribbled.

Janis spent one night in the hospital, but left before the doctors finished analyzing the results of the lymph node dissection. She and Chris drove straight to Cape Cod, their favorite retreat. They'd long thought about buying a condo there. It would probably be cheaper than all the hotel bills they racked up with their many trips out there. But it never seemed to be the right time for them, either financially or logistically.

That weekend, Janis got another call from her surgeon; by now, she was getting used to having important information delivered over the phone. This time it was all good news. All her lymph nodes were negative; there had been no discernible spreading. Janis and Chris were excited, and celebrated with a quiet dinner at their favorite Italian restaurant.

Treatment Choices

Next, Janis had to decide on a treatment plan. Her oncologist suggested radiation and chemotherapy, but Janis had reservations.

"I worry that this is the most toxic thing I can do to my body," Janis told Chris. "I've got to be certain that this is the right decision." Together, Janis and Chris cruised the Internet and perused bookstores and libraries. Janis called a few breast surgeons and breast cancer survivors to ask advice.

Finally, Janis felt she had enough information to make a decision. She decided she agreed with her oncologist. "The combination of radiation to treat the breast and chemotherapy to zap any lingering cancer cells elsewhere in my body is probably the best option Western medicine has to offer," she told Chris, patting her computer printouts and notes. "It can't be good for my body, but cancer is certainly worse."

Bike Helmet in Hand

Six and a half weeks of radiation came first. The treatments took an hour or more each day. Janis was determined not to succumb to the "I'm sick" mentality; she usually rode her bike around Boston's busy streets and she wasn't going to let cancer stop her routine. She walked into the clinic the way she walked into her office: carrying her helmet and her bike seat, much to the amusement and admiration of the doctors, nurses, and other patients.

Many radiation patients experience fatigue, but Janis never felt tired, even during the "booster" (or concentrated) treatments she received during the last week. Her breast was a little sore and she got what felt like a minor sunburn on the area during the last week, but it didn't slow her down. "You know what's really strange about all this?" she said. "Other than the actual treatments, I feel fine. I felt healthy before the diagnosis and I feel healthy now during treatment. It's bizarre that someone could even say I have breast cancer. It just doesn't make sense."

Janis did a lot of visualization during radiation. Several times a week, she sat quietly in her favorite rose-colored armchair and told herself that the radiation was eliminating any possible stray cancer cells. "I'm not sure if this is helping," she told Chris one evening as she made herself a cup of hot chocolate. "But it's always good to believe that the medicine you're receiving has some positive effect."

Working through the Chemo

Janis was terrified of the next phase of her treatment: chemotherapy. She didn't like the idea of having toxic chemicals coursing through her body. She hated what it looked like and hated the process of receiving it. Plus, she didn't want to lose her hair, she didn't want to feel sick, she didn't want to lose time from work; in short, she didn't want to change her whole life for chemotherapy.

So Janis took control of the things in her life she could control, outside of the chemo treatments. She continued to bike and work out at the gym several times a week, taking aerobics classes and lifting free weights. She tried meditation and yoga and increased the number of massages she received.

Many evenings, close friends came over carrying bags of groceries and containers of homemade macaroni and cheese, meatloaf, and mashed potatoes. They kicked Janis and Chris out of the kitchen as they measured, stirred, and reheated. After everyone ate, knocking elbows in the small dining room, Janis's friends retreated to the kitchen to clean up. Whenever Janis got up to help clear the table, Chris pulled her back into her chair. "It's hard work, letting people pamper you," Janis reflected.

Possibly the biggest change for Janis was learning to focus on herself. She cut back on her schedule, working only a five-day, forty-hour week. "Not being in the office all the time makes me feel like I'm giving up control," she explained to Chris. "That's hard to do." She had always been the one other staff members came to with questions or problems. She continued to lend a supportive ear, but found she was no longer offering to take care of last-minute details for others.

"I'm glad to hear it," said Chris. "You can't stay until eight *every* night."

After completing her chemotherapy treatment, Janis joined a support group for women with cancer at Fenway Community Health Center. Many, but not all, of the eight women had had breast cancer, and they ranged in age from late twenties to early fifties. Janis faithfully went to the facilitator-led weekly meetings. She sat quietly in one of the folding chairs that formed a circle. She felt that she had been through the worst of it and wanted to leave most of the hour-long session open for women still in treatment. But she appreciated listening to the other women's stories. "It makes me feel sad—and lucky—to know that other women have had worse experiences than me," she said. Perhaps even more important, the group showed her that she wasn't the only young woman dealing with a diagnosis of breast cancer. Janis also found that her "success story" inspired other women.

Redirecting Priorities

"Life after cancer is a little strange," Janis told Chris. She was cancer-free and hoped to remain that way. She went to her doctors' appointments and knew she was being watched closely, but she found it hard to give up the battle. She had gotten the diagnosis of disease, geared herself up to go through treatment, and had come out believing that she won the battle.

Janis has come to believe that we're only as strong as the circumstances we're dealt. "We don't realize our strength until we're put in a situation that tests it and forces us to find the inner strength we need."

She finds that she is more careful with her time now than she was before breast cancer. She is more concerned about setting priorities and trying to make time for things that are important to her. Fighting the disease showed her that she doesn't know how long her life is going to be; not that one ever knows, but all of a sudden, something that used to prompt an "I'll do it tomorrow" seems more urgent. Breast cancer helped her take stock of her life, helped her see that her relationships with friends and family are more important than working a few more hours a day. She realized that life is short, that she doesn't have a lot of time to waste, and that she doesn't want to spend her time with people who don't mean a lot to her.

This new perspective is especially reflected in Janis's attitude toward her work. Two and a half years after diagnosis, Janis changed jobs. "I can't stand all this pressure," Janis told Chris. "I wish there were a way I could spend more time with you and with my friends and family." She quit her job and found one that offered more fun and definitely less stress.

And yet, as much as Janis loves her new position, she finds that she's not as dedicated to work as she was before breast cancer. Although she sometimes feels guilty about leaving work when other people are still there, she's determined that she won't fall back into her old six-days-a-week pattern.

⟡

One afternoon, the phone rang in her apartment.

"I have some bad news for you," Janis's mother began. "It's Howard. He's passed away." While Janis had battled her breast cancer, her brother had contracted AIDS and finally succumbed to the disease.

"I can't believe I've lost a son," her mother continued. "It's not right for children to die before their parents; it just wasn't meant to be." Janis mumbled some reassuring words. Then her mother interrupted. "I know I wasn't there for you as much as you would have liked when you were diagnosed with breast cancer," she continued in a softer voice. "But I want you to know that I'm glad I still have one child left."

A Healthy New Balance
Despite her triumph over breast cancer, there is a new sadness in Janis now. She's not sure whether it stems from her experience with

breast cancer or from her brother's death. Or both. But she has come to realize that perhaps it's not so important to pin it down.

Instead, Janis channels her sadness to fuel her activism. She uses her theater manager experience to run benefit concerts for the Massachusetts Breast Cancer Coalition. She is also a founding member of the Silent Spring Institute, an offshoot of the MBCC, which funds research into the environmental causes of cancer in general. Her latest project is helping to fund a new documentary on breast cancer. On a personal level, she has worked very hard to convince women to do monthly breast self-exams. She tells them, "That's how I found my lump."

Janis had smoked cigarettes for a long time and had tried to quit many times, but always gone back. Breast cancer was a signal that she couldn't keep doing something that she knew to be destructive. "I want to be as healthy as possible," she said, stubbing out her last cigarette and tossing her last ashtray into the trash can.

Life after breast cancer, Janis decided, meant being kinder to her body and to herself. That meant eating better, relaxing more, and finding a healthier balance between work and the rest of her life.

Janis still works in entertainment management in Boston, but her hours are closer to nine to five these days. She and Chris have adopted a dog named Sophie and moved to Jamaica Plain, a multi-racial neighborhood full of parks for the three of them to explore. A year after Janis finished treatment, they bought a small condominium on Cape Cod. "Breast cancer has shown me that I don't have a lot of time to waste," she said. "I want to enjoy life now, not just wait for the future." Every chance they get, Janis and Chris take off Friday afternoon, pack a small bag of clothes and toiletries, pop Sophie in the back seat, and head up Route 6 to the Cape. Janis is now eleven years out from her initial diagnosis and remains cancer-free.

□ □ □

Janis is not unusual in her decision to set limits on her career as a result of her diagnosis. Roberta, too, found it necessary to claim more time for herself. She decided to restructure her career to reclaim her life, to pare down her eighty-plus hours a week to no more than sixty.

Similarly, some women decided to work less than full-time. During treatment, Dana chose to take a part-time job and Helen went on short-term disability, which allowed her to focus solely on getting better. Mary, too, stopped working during treatment. When she returned to nursing, it was on a part-time basis, to allow herself to focus on her own health and the fitness-oriented support group she founded in her area. Clearly, breast cancer confronts women with the need to rethink their career choices, including their work/life balance.

WHAT IF I THRIVE ON MY CAREER?

❧ Anne,* 27: Getting Back to Business

ANNE THRIVED ON CHALLENGE. Dynamic and ambitious in her career, she reveled in financial research and analysis. She loved to learn about different systems and to operate among a plethora of moving pieces, juggling deadlines and working with multiple constituencies in a fast-paced environment. Battling breast cancer only intensified her commitment to her career, propelling her through an Ivy League MBA program and into her dream job on Wall Street doing equity research.

Even before graduate school, when she was in Chicago working in finance for a French manufacturing firm, Anne dressed in urban high fashion: black pantsuits, heels, and never so much as a chipped nail. Her thick, long hair was cut in a shapely style, and she treated herself to highlights every so often to complement her skin tone. She described herself as "a trendy city girl." A gym rat, Anne also enjoyed tennis, going to the movies, dating, and checking out the hottest new restaurants. In her spare time, Anne was involved with the Starlight

*Not her real name

Children's Foundation, a nonprofit organization that grants wishes to terminally ill children.

At age twenty-seven, Anne could multi-task with the best of them. In the process of transitioning from the auditing branch of her firm over to mergers and acquisitions, the position she had her heart set on, she was also applying for MBA programs, studying for the GMAT, and preparing her application essays.

Then one night, resting in a hotel in Ohio where she was traveling for business, Anne felt a lump in her breast.

She decided not to call her doctor right away; she assumed the lump was stress-related. The possibility of breast cancer did not cross her mind. First she waited until she got her period to see if the lump was related to hormonal changes. Then she held off until after the GMAT. Getting into business school was her longtime dream and she didn't want anything to distract her. She hadn't told anyone about the lump, not even her mother, with whom she was very close.

"A Little Unusual"

Three months later, she finally went to see her gynecologist, the doctor who'd been checking Anne and her mother, Lisa, for years. He'd delivered Anne's brother, who was currently twenty-four years old.

The doctor gave Anne a manual breast exam and recommended a needle biopsy after feeling the lump. He didn't think it was anything to worry about, but thought it was better to be safe and check it out. He performed the needle biopsy right there in his office.

A few days later, Anne received a message from her doctor asking her to call him. She checked her caller ID and saw that he had tried to reach her several times that day. Anne knew something was up; she began to feel nervous.

When she called the doctor the following morning, the receptionist put her right through to the doctor. He said, "We got the results back and they're a little unusual. Could you come to the hospital immediately for an ultrasound?" She packed up everything on her desk, including her computer, and got into her car.

As soon as she left the office, Anne pulled out her cell phone and called her mother. As she dialed, Anne started to cry. When she began to recount the story, her mother interrupted and said, "Anne, I know."

Anne was stunned. She didn't know what response she had expected, but this certainly wasn't it. As it turned out, her mother had called the doctor that day with a question about herself, and during that conversation he had asked her to wish Anne good luck.

"Good luck with what?" Lisa had asked.

The doctor was surprised to hear that Anne hadn't told her mother what was going on, especially since he knew how close the two were. But he'd already broached the topic, so he knew he had to fill in the rest of the details.

At the time, Anne didn't think anything of it, since the doctor had known her all his life; later on, though, she was a little disappointed that the doctor hadn't told her the news first.

"Anne, come home first," suggested Lisa. "We'll go to the hospital together."

Much as she didn't want to worry her mother until she understood what was happening with her body, Anne was relieved that Lisa knew what was going on. They were very close, almost like best friends, and had kept no secrets from each other before. Anne was a little concerned that her mother would get too emotional; she knew this situation must be difficult for a mother to handle. But Lisa really came through for Anne, and seeing her mother so resilient helped Anne keep it together, too.

They went together to see the breast surgeon, who recommended an outpatient procedure to extract a piece of the lump and biopsy it. He believed that the mass was too large to remove without leaving Anne's breast deformed. They set up one appointment for the procedure and a second to discuss the results.

The day after the operation, Anne went back to her job. She couldn't just sit at home and worry about the diagnosis. She figured she would either be very nauseated or eat five million pounds of ice cream. She didn't want to do either one; plus, she enjoyed her work tremendously. She was in the middle of a major project and had a lot of the background information and details at the tips of her fingers; she didn't want to miss the opportunity to see this phase of a merger.

Anne worked every day and even went into work on the morning of the follow-up consultation. Both her parents went to the appointment with her. The breast surgeon checked her stitches first, then called her parents into his office. They sat around a large wooden table.

"It's definitive," he said to Anne. "You have breast cancer."

Anne shut down. She didn't cry, she didn't talk, she couldn't take in what was being said. Later, she found out that she had mucinous carcinoma, a rare form of cancer and particularly unusual in young women. According to her surgeon, the tumor was surrounded by mucus, so it was less likely to spread.

❧

That night, Anne called her supervisor and told him that she had breast cancer. She had decided that honesty was best and that the office needed to know what was going on. Her supervisor said, "Oh, I'm sorry, but will you still be able to join us for a conference call tomorrow?" Anne was appalled by his insensitivity and mentioned it to a friend at the company. From then on, her supervisor was more respectful and sensitive to her situation.

A Million Questions

Once Anne knew her diagnosis, she realized she could no longer ignore the issue; she had to start researching breast cancer. She approached the process like a business endeavor. She read books, surfed the Internet, and put together questions, creating a different list for each doctor: breast surgeon, radiologist, and plastic surgeon. She used a different-colored font for each list: red for the radiologist, and so on.

Now Anne had to choose a breast surgeon. Location was a major concern for her—she was already commuting an hour and a half each

way to work. The surgeon who diagnosed her was located in the sub-
urbs near her parents. But that would have meant another long drive.
Should she choose a team of doctors at a hospital near her apartment?
Should she try to find someone near her office? Anne decided to check
out several surgeons and get multiple opinions on how to proceed.

Selecting doctors, Anne found, was one of the most difficult parts
of the diagnosis. It seemed as though all the doctors had different
ideas about treatment. One surgeon told Anne she needed a mastectomy and chemotherapy and was going to lose all her hair. Another
told her she probably only needed a lumpectomy, but he couldn't be
sure until he saw the lump itself, at which point he might determine
that she would need a mastectomy. If there were lymph nodes
involved, it would become even more complicated.

Ultimately, Anne picked a surgeon near her apartment in Chicago,
which would make treatment easier logistically. He was very frank
with her and had a pleasant bedside manner. He recommended a
lumpectomy, but Anne wasn't sure that was the right choice for her.
With a lumpectomy, radiation is required. Anne went to see a radiologist to discuss the radiation process. The radiologist was concerned
about the side effects of radiation on a twenty-seven-year-old woman.
"I can't tell you for sure what the long-term side effects will be
because there just haven't been enough studies of the effects of radiation in young women."

"So what happens if I get lung cancer as a result of the radiation?"
Anne mused. "I'm going to hate myself if I chose vanity over a more
severe surgery."

Ultimately, Anne decided on a mastectomy. She had always
believed in "no pain, no gain."

To complicate matters, Anne had been in the process of finding a
new apartment before all of this occurred. She'd signed a lease on a
new place in her current neighborhood just before she got the diagnosis, and her current lease was due to expire. She scheduled her
move for five days before the surgery, realizing that she had to do it
while she was still physically up to the challenge, before she was

weakened by surgery. It would drive her crazy if she couldn't carry a single box and had to sit on the sofa directing traffic. Anne organized her friends to help, which was a very unusual step for her. One friend packed up her kitchen, another did the closet, a third focused on the living room.

Just One Option

As it turned out, the surgical decision wasn't really Anne's to make. Her tumor was approximately four centimeters in diameter, about the size of a golf ball. Because it was so big, she would have needed a mastectomy anyway, so by deciding not to have a lumpectomy initially, she saved herself from having to undergo a second surgery.

As Anne recuperated in her hospital room, it was good to know that the cancer had been excised with clean margins. But she was still waiting to hear about her pathology report. One evening, when her parents and best friend were visiting, the surgeon came in with the report. "Great news: You have no lymph node involvement."

The whole family was euphoric; her prognosis had just improved radically. Anne tossed her thick hair in delight.

"But, Anne," the doctor added, "you'll need chemo."

She was devastated. "I didn't care about the cancer, I didn't care about getting better, I just didn't want to lose my hair," she told me.

After the surgery, Anne took two weeks off from work because her arm was too sore from the procedure to make the three-hour round-trip drive to the office. During this time, she stayed with her parents and visited with family and friends who stopped by to check up on her. She kept track of the gifts to write thank-you notes and realized she received about a hundred, not to mention flowers worthy of a garden at Versailles. She made a composite photograph of all the flowers she received. It still hangs in a frame in her current apartment, to remind her of how supportive her friends and family were during that difficult period.

A few days after surgery, Anne started feeling antsy. She was sore, but not in a lot of pain. "I don't want to sit home," she told her mother. "Let's go." So they went shopping, enjoying a little "retail therapy" and having a nice lunch out.

At this point, Anne started to hear back from business schools. She didn't get into any of her top picks. It was a big disappointment, but Anne took it in stride. Things happen for a reason, she told herself, so now she was able to focus on treatment and getting healthy.

Going for her first checkup was also disheartening. The doctor asked her to raise both of her hands over her head and she couldn't. "I thought I'd never be able to work out again."

The thought of seeing the oncologist terrified Anne. "The only thing I could picture was the movie *Dying Young*: Everyone was completely emaciated, bald, looking deathly ill." She sat on her parents' living room couch and cried. She remembered talking to one survivor who told her, "I gained twenty pounds, lost all my hair, and quit my job." Anne was sure her life was over. "I'm going to have to stay home, I'm going to have to change jobs, I'm not going to be able to work out, I'm going to gain twenty pounds," she wailed. "It's horrible."

Lisa was so worried about her daughter that she called the oncologist, whom Anne had only met once. He reassured Lisa that the scenario Anne had envisioned wasn't necessarily going to happen.

Anne received chemotherapy once a month, and although her hair did thin out somewhat, she didn't lose it all. And she didn't quit her job; if anything, she catapulted herself into an even more influential position as her superiors at work had been impressed with her ability to remain strong and balance her medical treatment and work life.

Telecommuting

When Anne was ready to go back to work, she set some clear limits with her supervisor. "I will be having chemo once a month and I commute an hour and a half to work every day. I'm going to work from home on Fridays and Mondays for a while." She explained that the change wouldn't get in the way of her job. "I have a fax at home, I have a cell phone, and I have a computer with remote e-mail." He agreed. She was pleased with her own ability to take charge of the situation and manage it to meet her needs.

Other than working at home a few days a week, Anne didn't let chemotherapy interrupt her life any more than her surgery had. Driven to excel, she continued to work sixty hours a week and continued going to the gym two or three times a week, often straight from chemotherapy treatment. She had gained twenty pounds from the steroids and felt she had to do something about that. Plus, exercise made her feel better about herself.

But life didn't get completely back to normal. The first time she went to the grocery store, she had some friends come along to carry the bags. She had a hard time hailing a cab because she couldn't lift her hand high enough. Chemotherapy itself wasn't fatiguing until about the fifth or sixth month. But even then, the fatigue wasn't debilitating; it felt more like jet lag.

Anne met a new man in a bar two months after she started chemotherapy, the night before she was planning to do a breast cancer walk with her family. They sat sipping drinks and talked until about three in the morning. She didn't mention breast cancer or chemotherapy.

After a few dates, she told him what was going on. She wanted to be honest and he was the first person she had dated since her diagnosis. At the time, he was supportive, but shortly after she told him, he stopped calling. He provided no explanation.

Eventually, Anne decided to confront him and try to find out what happened. She called and said, "I need to know why you stopped calling me. We travel in the same circles, I'm sure I'm going to run into you and I don't want to be angry with you. I want us to be friends. But I need to know why you stopped talking to me." She wanted to ask him if it was because of her breast cancer, but was afraid to be that explicit; she couldn't trust that he would answer her honestly. "It's just that I'm not over an ex-girlfriend," he said. "I'm not ready to date right now." But Anne was never convinced by that explanation, she was never really sure what happened.

꿏

When the surgeon performed the mastectomy on her left breast, he inserted a tissue expander, which was later filled with saline to reconstruct the breast. At the same time, Anne had her right breast reduced from a size D down to a B. "I've always, always had problems with my breasts, like with running." But she never would have had the breast reduction if she weren't already having breast surgery.

In February and March, Anne wore big sweaters. By summer, she was able to go back to the gym, she started lying out in the sun, and she bought new bikinis to fit her now-smaller bosom.

To celebrate finishing chemo, Anne and her mother went to a spa for four luxurious days. Anne enjoyed being pampered with massages, facials, saunas, and participating in cooking, nutrition, and yoga classes. She figured her body had just experienced a traumatic period and deserved to be pampered.

Upon returning from her spa trip, Anne got right back into the swing of things, working hard at her job and filling out her graduate school applications. To reapply to the Wharton School of Business at the University of Pennsylvania, she was required to write an essay about what she had done over the past year that would make her a stronger candidate. "This will be easy for me, I certainly have a lot to write about," she told Lisa, who diligently read each essay. "I'll just write about what I went through, and what I've learned from the past year."

Continuing Education

Business school was everything Anne had hoped for, though nothing like what she had envisioned. What really stood out about the MBA program was the relationships she built at Wharton. "I entered a network of eight hundred people from around the world, all about the same age and the same intellectual level. I built an amazing network of friends and career colleagues."

Studying at Wharton was particularly demanding for Anne because she decided to keep quiet about her breast cancer. This was quite a change for her, because back in Chicago, everyone knew. Friends warned Anne that she could never be fully open in an interview because it was hard to know whether a company would discriminate because of her cancer history. Anne fiercely wanted a job on Wall Street and she worried about the competition, especially because the economy was starting to slow at that time. She didn't want to take any chances. She didn't want anyone to know that she had had breast cancer.

Anne didn't want people to see her as different. She didn't want friends or colleagues to baby her, treat her differently, or feel sorry for her. That was not her style. But this discretion was difficult for Anne. Relationships, she found, were tricky when she was hiding something, especially something as important as breast cancer. She hated to be so shielded.

Anne got a summer internship at an investment banking firm on Wall Street and worked long, long hours.

"This is the job I coveted, the reason I went to grad school," she told me. "I worked very hard to get it. The competition was steep. And I was very lucky. I love what I do, I love the people I work with. This summer internship has confirmed that I really want to do equity research full time."

After graduating from Wharton, she landed a dream job at another Wall Street investment bank, also in equity research, starting that upcoming fall. After a summer of travel in East Asia, Anne moved to the Big Apple, to a one-bedroom apartment in Manhattan.

"Think about it, Mom: After breast cancer, after grad school, after all that, I'm exactly where I wanted to be. Maybe even ahead," Anne rejoiced one afternoon.

"I'm very proud of you. You really learned how to deal with adversity," Lisa said. "But I am still worried about the number of hours you work."

"Working sixty-plus hours a week is not bad," Anne explained to her mother. She coped by not trying to do everything herself. "I have my apartment cleaned, I don't cook, I don't go to the grocery store, and I have my clothing dry-cleaned." And she worked hard at trying to figure out the balance in her life: juggling time with friends, time with family, time at work, and at least a couple of hours of sleep every night.

A Second Diagnosis

At one year into the job, more than three and a half years after being diagnosed with breast cancer, Anne felt that her life was stable. She wasn't changing apartments, she wasn't looking for a job, and she wasn't in a tumultuous position. She had great friends and family.

And then, almost exactly four years after her initial diagnosis, Anne was diagnosed with metastasized bone and lung cancer.

Her breast cancer wasn't supposed to spread, her doctors had told her, but it did. The doctors started Anne on antihormonal treatment to stop her estrogen flow; the medication put her, functionally, in menopause. The treatment controls the cancer, but doctors can't cure it. "As long as the tumors are shrinking and are contained and not spreading, you're fine," her doctors assured her. That will continue as long as the medicine keeps working. "How long the medicine is going to keep working, we don't know," the doctors said. Every few months Anne has CAT and bone scans and gets an injection to stop her estrogen flow.

For Anne, the worst part was the hot flashes. At age thirty-two, it was hard to have her body behave as though she were fifty-five. It was hard to go to a crowded bar on a Saturday night; she often found herself sweating. But she didn't let that stop her from going in the first place. If she felt uncomfortable, she'd just leave, knowing she had given it a good try.

Staying Up to Speed

Her second diagnosis of cancer changed Anne's attitude toward sharing her story. She sent out a long, descriptive e-mail to nearly a hundred friends, including many people from business school who hadn't known about her past experience with breast cancer. She didn't want rumors to go flying; she wanted to tell the truth in her own words. The e-mail explained her diagnosis, treatment, and prognosis.

"I don't want you to treat me any differently," she wrote. "I don't want you to say 'Anne has more problems than anyone else so I can't tell her about breaking up with my boyfriend.' I still want you to keep treating me as a confidante. I want to remind everyone that it takes two to tango and I want all of you to remember that I am also here for you—as you have been for me. When you need an ear, an arm, or just a friend to hang with, I am here."

Anne also decided to tell her supervisor, Carol. She reasoned, "In this economy, I can't be going to the doctor that frequently or people will get suspicious. I don't think I could hide it. And if I'm going to tell them I'm sick, I might as well tell them what's going on. It makes no sense to be secretive. Honesty and candor are important to me."

Carol was extremely sensitive and supportive. Every time Anne went to the doctor, Carol asked how it went and how she felt. Anne asked Carol not to treat her specially. "I want you to pretend as though nothing's wrong with me. Because if you treat me as though there's something wrong, then we're going to be very inefficient. We're not going to be productive. You're constantly going to worry about how to manage me, what work to give me, et cetera. I want the onus to be on me. If I can't handle something and I have too much on my plate, I have to be the one to speak up."

Carol nodded.

"At the same time, if I'm not performing up to speed, you have to be able to tell me. Otherwise, I might as well not be here."

That little speech stood her in good stead. That summer, six months after her second diagnosis, work slowed down and Anne confronted Carol. "Are you going easy on me?" she asked.

"No. It's a timing matter," Carol responded. "That's how Wall Street works. There are high points and low points. Take advantage of the slow time and enjoy it. Trust me, when it gets crazy, you're going to wish you had this time again. It comes in waves."

Survivor Suggestions on Taking Care of Your Self

☐ Reward yourself throughout your treatment, you deserve it. Rewards can be tangible items, special dinners, vacations—whatever gives you pleasure and comfort.

☐ Learn to be selfish.

☐ Take care of your body; take care of your soul.

☐ Learn to forgive people—including yourself.

☐ Give yourself permission to feel sad. It's okay to cry.

☐ Give yourself mini-vacations during treatment.

☐ Allow yourself to have fun. Don't just sit at home if that's not your style.

☐ Being careful about your health is not the same as hypochondria; after cancer, you *should* be careful.

☐ Don't indulge in self-pity.

☐ Realize and appreciate your own strengths.

Carol was right. Shortly after that conversation, the pace at work picked up and Anne took the lead in a new project. She was eager for the challenge, not because she wanted distraction from the cancer, but because she was finally able to pursue her goal of being an equity research analyst on Wall Street.

Business as Usual

Anne doesn't think her go-getting attitude toward work stems from the cancer diagnosis. She was just as resolute about her career before she found the lump.

"I'm just not a 'sit around' person," said Anne. "I am ambitious and invested in my career. I love that I'm constantly learning more and becoming more educated."

Anne makes sure she has time to see friends and to go to the theater and the movies and to take vacations. She puts time and energy into her career because she loves her job and is thrilled to take on a challenge. She would love to have a relationship and a husband, but feels she has worked too hard and come too far to take the focus off her career.

"I don't view my diagnoses as life-destructive experiences, but I realize how I've drawn on a deeper part of myself, how eager I am to flourish in the future," Anne said. "I'm ready to enter the next phase of my life and promote my passion and commitment to learning new things. I've become a very strong, independent person who has demonstrated in my own life that a difficult experience can be a challenge, but it can also be conquered with success. If anything, fighting cancer has made me *more* confident and strong."

Anne continues to work in equity research on Wall Street. Her career is flourishing. She is in treatment for her bone and lung cancer. The drugs that she is taking all seem to be working to contain the cancer. It is not curable, but the cancer has shrunk and is not spreading—and that, she says, is the best that she can ask for.

◻ ◻ ◻

Anne is not the only woman to find that her career was an area that she could control, a source of comfort during the unpredictability of breast cancer treatment. But it is difficult to become immersed in a career without a supportive supervisor and a flexible work environment. Roberta and Amanda both enjoyed these benefits. Roberta was able to work from home and Amanda's company let her work out of another regional office while she was out of town for radiation treatment. As a result, both women put a lot of energy into their career.

Other women were not able to continue working. Insurance difficulties forced Nora out of the workplace, whereas Becky's dance career was waylaid by the physical limitations of breast cancer treatment. Both returned to their careers with even greater enthusiasm as soon as they were economically and physically able.

WHAT IF I HAVE NO HEALTH INSURANCE?

✺ Nora,* 27: Adventures in Medicaid

NORA ENJOYED THE WORK AND THE GLAMOUR of creating music videos and films. She could rouse a New York sidestreet out of its dawn slumber to make it bustle like midtown at rush hour, transform autumnal leaves into winter snowdrifts, and gentrify questionable neighborhoods to fool a camera's eye. When she went to the art-house movie theater to see the latest hit or catch a preview for the industry, she could often match a face with many of the behind-the-scenes names. She enjoyed both the physical and artistic components to set design. And she thrilled over the fun and fast pace of it all.

At twenty-seven, Nora loved the freelance lifestyle. She thrived on working seventeen hours straight, fueled by coffee, candy, cigarettes, and catered meals. After a long day, she'd go home and sleep for six hours, then return to the set and transform it again. The forced vacations between projects weren't bad, either. This lifestyle didn't seem to take a toll on her five-foot-seven, slender body, topped with a head of wavy blond hair. She never got a cold and was in great physical shape. And she never had to work at it.

Living in Williamsburg, a vibrant and artsy neighborhood in Brooklyn, Nora was far from her family. Her parents, with whom she had shaky relationships, lived in the coastal city of Wilmington, North Carolina. Her three brothers, with whom she rarely spoke, lived in Atlanta and Washington, D.C.

*Not her real name

She just couldn't imagine what her life would be like without having her work to define it. Until she had to give up her job and go on welfare to get health insurance to pay for breast cancer treatment.

✦❦✦

One September, Nora met Mark at a party. He was six feet, three inches tall and in good physical shape. Her longtime friend, Elizabeth, had set Nora up, as she had several times in the past. But this was the first match to click.

For their first date, they went to a film, then had late-night sushi. As they sat eating California rolls in a small, dimly lit restaurant, Nora was struck by how much they had in common. They both worked in film—Mark did technical work, mostly in music videos—and they both liked the same foods, sushi in particular.

Mark introduced Nora to motorcycle riding. Staring at his black Harley, Nora was nervous; how was such a tiny machine going to hold them both? But after their first ride around Manhattan, weaving through the traffic on the FDR Drive as she held tight to Mark, Nora was hooked. After a week and a half of dating, Nora bought herself a motorcycle helmet.

No sooner had Nora realized that she was falling in love with the tall, auburn-haired man then everything changed. Mark and Nora were sitting in Nora's sparsely decorated apartment, on her grandmother's gold-upholstered sofa, kissing. Mark slipped his hand up Nora's V-neck sweater and stroked her breasts.

"Hey," Mark said gently. "Do you know you have a lump?"

"Oh my God! Do I?" Nora gasped. She didn't say her next thought out loud, but she could only come up with one explanation for a lump in a breast.

Nora hadn't been to a gynecologist in a long time, partly because her freelance work didn't provide health insurance and partly because it didn't provide much free time. But she'd just gotten a generous check from her grandfather. She decided to splurge on a gynecological checkup.

A Rude Awakening

While Nora waited for the day of the appointment, she surfed the Internet and decided she had a fibroadenoma. A benign lump, nothing to worry about.

On the appointed day, Nora took an early lunch break and went to the gynecologist. The doctor analyzed her gynecological history. When he heard that her periods weren't regular, he said, "You probably have polycystic ovarian syndrome. That causes irregular periods. You'll need birth control pills to treat that. Otherwise, polycystic ovarian syndrome can cause infertility."

"What about the lump in my breast?" Nora asked.

"You might have breast cancer," he said. "You should see a breast surgeon."

Nora was disappointed that he was unable to tell her whether she had cancer or a fibroadenoma and disturbed that it didn't seem to bother him. Nora decided to see one of the best, and therefore busiest, breast surgeons in New York. She had to wait two weeks for an appointment. To keep her mind off of her health, she focused on Mark. She pushed aside occasional moments of anxiety, still believing she had a fibroadenoma. She took birth control pills for her polycystic ovarian syndrome and convinced herself she was going to be fine.

The breast surgeon suggested that Nora have the lump biopsied and he scheduled an appointment for three days later. Although Nora wasn't close to her family, her parents were very supportive once she told them about the lump. Her father, David, a college professor, found someone to teach his classes and flew in from North Carolina. Her mother, Joan, was unreachable, on a business trip in Poland. Nora called all three of her brothers the night before the surgery. She just wanted them to know what was going on and she shared the bare minimum. "I'm having a biopsy of my left breast. It's very minor. I'm probably fine," she told them.

Mark went to the hospital along with her father. Just before the appointment, Nora and Mark excused themselves and made love quickly and desperately in the handicapped bathroom. For Nora, sex wasn't just hot and steamy—it felt life-affirming at a time she needed it most.

When Nora awoke after the surgery, she became aware of conversation around her.

"It was malignant," the breast surgeon was saying. Nora heard the words, but they made no impression.

"Is she going to die?" David asked. While hearing the diagnosis in her doctor's voice didn't affect her, hearing the fear in her father's voice was truly disturbing. Someone had finally reached her mother, who had flown directly to New York from Europe. Joan was standing quietly in the room, her gaze fixed on her daughter.

"We don't know yet," the surgeon responded. "It doesn't look that advanced. We're going to have the lab look at it and then we'll know more."

When the family returned to Nora's apartment, David became a blur of activity. He rummaged through her kitchen cabinets. "You need milk, you need soup," he said as he hurried out the front door of the second-floor apartment. He returned about fifteen minutes later with plastic bags holding a half-gallon of 2 percent milk and a couple of cans of chicken noodle soup. He looked in her bathroom. "You don't have enough toilet paper," he said, ignoring the five rolls Nora had stored in the cabinet. He hurried out the door again. Once the shopping was done, David blew up the air mattress he had bought for himself and Joan to sleep on. He was puffing into it as Nora walked into her bedroom. When she came back into the living room, she found him holding the mattress in his hands, staring out the window at the sky, perfectly still. As she looked at her father's broad face—for once expressionless, still and quiet—she realized the gravity of the situation. What she couldn't see in herself she read in her father's face.

Family and Friends Respond

Not only did Nora feel angry, scared, and saddened by her diagnosis of breast cancer, she felt ashamed as well. She thought breast cancer was a sex-specific disease and worried that people wouldn't take it seriously. "My college friend had a brain tumor," she said, "and everyone knows how dangerous that is; no one takes breast cancer seriously." Nora saw breast cancer as a feminine weakness. And so did a lot of her friends, who simply didn't realize that breast cancer is a life-threatening disease. Even her gynecologist initially told her, "Worst-case scenario, you lose a breast."

She realized that this attitude affects the political arena as well. There has been less funding available, historically, for breast cancer research than for most other forms of cancer research. Indeed, the federal government has, at times, considered cutting the funding altogether.

That sense of shame made it even more difficult to tell people.

Gerry, Nora's older brother by three years, called her apartment twenty minutes after Nora and her parents got back from the hospital.

"Hey, N."

"Hey, G, what's up?"

"How was the surgery? Everything okay?"

Nora handed the telephone to her father and walked out of the room. She could not bring herself to say the words out loud; even hearing her father relate the diagnosis was terrifying. Nora heard her father name the disease and begin to cry. That was the last time for months that she tried to tell someone that she had breast cancer. She asked Joan to call Mark and then spread the word to relatives.

The next evening, Mark and Nora took a cab to a club in the East Village to hear one of Nora's favorite bands. Nora snuggled with Mark in the backseat, wanting to *feel* his support. Then she leaned over to kiss him. Mark and Nora had sex in the cab, completely sober. Sex just made Nora feel more alive, more her old self. It was one of the few things that did.

✿

Nora eventually found the courage to tell a few friends, but she found that she couldn't handle the way people responded. Reactions ranged from supportive to puzzling to out-and-out negative. For instance, after the initial appointment with the gynecologist, Nora called her friend Elizabeth. Nora was very upset, and Elizabeth was reassuring. After the biopsy, however, Elizabeth never called to check in. Finally, three days after she got the results, Nora called her. They exchanged greetings, then Nora broke the news.

"Elizabeth, I have breast cancer."

Her friend's call waiting beeped in.

"Hey, can you hold on?" Elizabeth asked.

"Sure," Nora said, feeling hurt.

Thirty seconds later, Elizabeth's live-in boyfriend got on the phone and said, "Listen, can Elizabeth call you back?"

Nora thought for a moment, then said, "You know, she doesn't need to call me back. Yes, that's it, tell Elizabeth *not* to call me back."

Mark later told her that *he* had made the interrupting call and that it hadn't been particularly important; he just wanted the name of a nearby restaurant that delivered egg sandwiches.

Others were terrified by Nora's diagnosis. Like Nora, her friends thought they were invincible. Then Nora got breast cancer. That wasn't supposed to happen yet, not for another twenty or thirty years. One friend avoided all phone calls and literally stopped speaking to Nora. Another friend called regularly, always inquiring about her health and sounding concerned; he would set a time to get together, but always canceled just as Nora was about to walk out the door.

⁂

Nora got the full biopsy report a week after her diagnosis. Not only was the lump malignant, but the cancer had also spread to one lymph node. The cancer cells were reproducing rapidly. She was going to need either a lumpectomy and radiation or a mastectomy. Either way, she would need chemotherapy treatment to prevent the cancer cells from spreading.

Lining Things Up

Nora realized, with a sick feeling in her stomach, that she had to find a way to pay for all of this medical care—the diagnostic tests, the surgery, the pending treatment. Nora was a freelancer, and thus had no medical insurance through an employer. How was she going to handle the medical bills without insurance?

At her breast surgeon's suggestion, she applied for Medicaid, using the hospital's Medicaid extension office. Having grown up in what she called the "upper-middle class," Nora never thought she would be dependent upon government assistance. She just never cared about having or making a lot of money. She was relieved to have medical coverage—she was eligible for the program—but she was embarrassed about being in a position where she needed that kind of help. "Great, just great," Nora thought. "One day I'm a freelancer, the next I'm a freeloader."

To receive Medicaid, however, Nora was forced to stop working. So, one week after diagnosis, Nora quit her freelance career to focus on getting better.

꿈

Mastectomy or lumpectomy? That was the hardest decision she had ever faced. Nora researched both options exhaustively, both on the Internet and at a nearby medical library. After hours of reading, she realized that nobody knew very much about breast cancer, especially in young women. The treatments, particularly chemotherapy, seemed so severe. She found it hard to believe she couldn't walk down to the pharmacy, spend twelve bucks, and be done with this in a week. She was going to be sick for a long time, something she'd never experienced before. Nora was disgusted with what the medical profession didn't know about breast cancer, terrified of what they did know, and horrified at the treatments available. She viewed mastectomy as mutilation, a procedure developed by male doctors who didn't know or care what it felt like to lose a breast. She opted for a lumpectomy.

The next decision was to select a chemotherapy regimen. The first oncologist Nora saw told her that her survival rate would be 65 percent with chemotherapy treatment, because of the speed at which the cancer cells were reproducing. He recommended she receive extremely high doses of drugs and performed some tests to determine how much her heart could handle. He told her that she should get blood donations from her family in case she needed a blood transfusion. And he enumerated the possible side effects: leukemia, infertility, and hospitalization at the end of almost every treatment. This regimen was her only chance to beat the cancer, the doctor emphasized. Nora worried that if she didn't die of the cancer—or the treatment—she would certainly be sickly for the rest of her life.

So she went back to the library. Nora kept reading until she realized that she wasn't finding anything new. She decided to seek out other opinions. The second oncologist Nora saw explained that because of her age and the fact that the cancer had already spread to one lymph node, selecting the most effective chemotherapy regimen was a hard call. His recommendation was that she do the less rigorous regimen because she was so young and wouldn't want to put her body through the stress of the more rigorous one.

The third oncologist agreed with the second, and Nora decided to stick with him. She felt very good about him; he sometimes appeared in her dreams. She found him very friendly, very gregarious, and, most important, very honest. When Nora brought in a question, he would take it seriously. He would fold his arms, step back to the wall, and say, "This is what we know, this is what we don't know.... The studies aren't definitive, we don't really know.... This is my gut feeling, but that's really all it is. You need to make your own decision."

Nora got her second and third opinions before Medicaid kicked in, wiping out her bank account. She decided that it was more important to treat the cancer than to avoid debt.

One evening, a week or two after her diagnosis, Nora was taking a bubble bath and thinking about her mortality. Just then, Dorian Gray, Nora's red-and-white longhaired cat, walked into the bathroom and sat down next to the tub. He had lived with her for the four years she'd been in this apartment. He lifted his back paw up to his mouth and began to groom himself. Watching Dorian made Nora remember Grace, her college friend who had just died of a brain tumor. During Grace's wake, at her parents' home, Grace's cat had been chasing a small red ball.

Nora wondered which of them would live longer: her or Dorian Gray?

Recuperating on the Beach

The lumpectomy was followed by six months of chemotherapy treatment, which were unlike anything Nora had ever experienced. Before breast cancer, she had no aversion to needles—it never bothered her to get shots or give blood—but after chemotherapy, they made her nauseated. "Classical Pavlovian conditioning," she told Mark.

Nora received chemotherapy treatments every three weeks. The chemicals pervaded Nora's entire body. They left a sweet, metallic taste in her mouth and she could feel them coursing through her bloodstream. She was simultaneously exhausted and wide awake; she was worn out, but her mind kept churning and she needed sleeping pills to take even a brief nap.

Her chemo experience was made worse by the anti-nausea steroid. It did its job (she rarely vomited), but it made her depressed and agitated. Her doctors made her take the medication because they were concerned that she might drop more weight from her already slender frame.

After each treatment, Nora needed help with day-to-day chores such as dressing, bathing, and preparing food. She hadn't been very close to her mother before the diagnosis, but during treatment, Joan, and sometimes David, came up to New York for almost every chemo session and stayed for three or four days. They did Nora's laundry, stocked her refrigerator, and cooked pots of pasta dishes and thick soups. Joan and Nora sat and talked for hours on the bed, reminiscing, discussing the unfairness of life, and catching up on family gossip. In between treatments, Nora went to her parents' home in North Carolina for about a week. They would walk along Wrightsville Beach or stroll the streets of historic downtown Wilmington. Whenever they were apart, Joan and Nora spoke every few days. For the first time in years, they fit their roles: Nora was the daughter needing help and her mother gave it freely.

Nora's body changed, of course, during chemotherapy treatment. Her normally milkmaid skin broke out incessantly and her previously thick blond hair grew very thin. In addition, because Nora was nauseated most of the time and because the only way to overcome the nausea was to eat, she gained ten pounds. She felt like she was the ugliest person in the world.

Not only was Nora bombarded with all of these physical symptoms, but she was also depressed. She was afraid of dying. She was exhausted. Because she wasn't working, she had little to focus on other than being sick. Because she was depressed, she didn't *want* to do anything. She and Mark broke up near the end of her chemotherapy treatment. "This is too difficult and too sad for me," he told her. "My father died of lung cancer three years ago. I can't look at you without thinking I'm going to lose you, too." Nora didn't know how to respond; it was too hard for her, too.

Nora wasn't financially independent anymore. Her parents paid her rent and plane fare so she could go to North Carolina for visits and covered most of her living expenses; Medicaid took care of the medical bills. It was heartening to know that her family cared and was willing to help, but she was uncomfortable about being so dependent.

Looking to the future was frightening as well. Nora knew that when she was finished with treatment, when she could return to a career, she would have to find a new one; her post-chemo body just wouldn't be able to handle the physical demands of film work. She took classes in desktop publishing, hoping that might be the career for her, but found it a little boring.

Most disturbing was the change in Nora's sense of self. She felt as though she had just started creating who she was, she had just started building a life for herself. And then she was diagnosed with breast cancer and that stripped away her identity. She simply didn't feel as though she had anything substantial in her life. "Being a sick person," she told her friends, "isn't much of a role to play when you're twenty-seven."

Nora did have one outlet, a high school friend who lived in New Mexico. They talked every month or so, and Nora told her about how chemo made her almost too tired to breathe and how she was afraid to go to sleep some nights. Nora really appreciated these conversations, but never shared the thoughts with anyone else.

Little White Specks

After Nora finished six months of chemo, she was scheduled for radiation treatment. She went in to the hospital for a routine checkup, including a mammogram. After the mammogram, Nora went back to the waiting room to see if the test had come out clearly enough. "Jeez, it's taking a long time," she thought.

Then they called Nora back to the exam room. Her mammogram film was hanging on the wall on top of the light box. She saw the little white specks that looked like flecks of dust on the film. "Oh my gosh," Nora said, sucking in her breath.

"How do you know what it is?" the radiologist asked.

"I've been doing this for six months. I recognize the calcifications." Nora closed her eyes for a moment. "How soon can you do the biopsy?" she asked, aware that calcifications are sometimes, but not always, a sign of cancer.

"We can schedule you in two weeks," the radiologist said, checking his clipboard.

"But I'm supposed to start radiation next week," Nora said, feeling a little frantic. "Can't you do it any sooner?"

"Well," he said, looking back at his clipboard. "We can do it in twenty minutes."

"Okay, then. Twenty minutes."

Nora was terrified. She had less than a half hour to prepare for the possibility of recurrence. *This* time, she knew what she was in for; she remembered the physical pain, she understood the disruptions to her life. And she knew that having a recurrence so quickly hurt her chances of survival. She was more scared now than she had been when she found the initial lump. The thought of going through chemotherapy again was even more disturbing than the idea that the cancer had returned.

When they started the procedure, Nora was nauseated and alternately cold and sweating. She perched precariously on a stool to raise her up to the machine that would extract the cells from her breast.

They found more cancer.

Taking No Chances

Nora decided that she wanted a mastectomy this time. Not another lumpectomy. "Take it all off," she told the surgeon. She didn't want to take any chances. But this decision was more difficult; it was hard to reconcile losing a breast. Nora cried for three weeks.

She called Mark. "This is not how I wanted to be calling you," she began, "but I need to get back the money I loaned you."

"Well, sure, but why? I thought you didn't need it right away."

"I have to pay for some surgery. I've had a recurrence of the breast cancer."

Nora heard Mark suck in his breath. When he asked, "Can I come over?" his voice was softer, more concerned.

Mark came to her apartment. They talked. And snuggled. By the end of the evening, they had decided to get back together. As nervous about intimacy as Nora felt, it was warm and comfortable in Mark's arms.

Alternative Therapy

She had her mastectomy a week and a half later, on a Monday morning. The recuperation was very painful and she took as much morphine as the surgeon would approve, more than usually allowed. It hurt to move; she couldn't breathe normally; it almost hurt to think.

The plastic surgeon wanted to make sure Nora looked at her chest before she left the hospital. She wanted Nora to be prepared for her new body.

"Hello, beautiful," the surgeon's nurse said in a cheery voice. "Come on, let's see you. Let's have you have a look at this thing. It's not so bad, you'll see." She took off the bandages, helped Nora sit up on her bed, and held a mirror in front of her chest. Nora pushed it away at first, then reached for it and stared. "It's not so bad," she told the nurse. "It's just the shock of seeing my breast gone."

After the mastectomy, Joan came to stay for a week. Mark was around to help, too, mostly by taking her mind off the mastectomy. He told her stories about work, about his other friends, about the latest movies and bands he'd seen. Nora found it was a relief *not* to talk about breast cancer.

Four days after the operation, that Friday night, she rode on the back of Mark's motorcycle from her Brooklyn apartment into Manhattan, to see an off-Broadway show. She hugged him tightly but cautiously so as not to aggravate her bandages. They enjoyed the show, though Nora was careful not to laugh too hard; her usual hearty laughter hurt her chest.

Nora didn't have chemotherapy after her recurrence because the cancer was in scar tissue, which was removed by the mastectomy. The oncologist determined that the cancer probably hadn't traveled out of her left breast. Nevertheless, he put Nora on a quarterly checkup schedule, instead of the typical biannual exams. Nora started her own preventive care: She began to exercise regularly, take essiac (an anticarcinogenic herb), and stick to a low-fat diet.

Around this time, Nora found out that she did not have polycystic ovarian syndrome; she never had. The doctor had never tested her for the disease; he simply assumed it because her periods were irregular. She also learned that birth control pills, which the gynecologist had prescribed for the polycystic ovarian syndrome, aggravate breast cancer and may have contributed to the fast rate at which her cancer cells had been dividing.

🖎

Two years after her diagnosis, Nora decided to try the anticancer drug tamoxifen, because her cancer had been estrogen-receptive. The side effects were more than she could handle. Hot flashes, light menstrual periods, volatile emotions around her periods. "I'm PMS-ing like a crazy woman," she told her mother. She read the technical research articles about tamoxifen and realized that none of the studies had looked at even a single woman under age thirty-five. It wasn't at all clear that the data about older women would also apply to her. "I wish they did more research on young women," she told her mother. So Nora stopped taking the drug. It wasn't worth enduring the side effects without some assurance that the drug would improve her chances of survival.

Working with Clearer Priorities

To her surprise, surviving breast cancer granted Nora more confidence and more drive. After breast cancer, she doesn't care if someone doesn't like her, she doesn't care whether what she does bothers someone, and she doesn't care if people think she's stepping on their toes. She is clearer about her priorities. "If someone insults me," she explained, "I call them on it. I don't just sit back and let someone treat me unfairly."

But that doesn't mean that Nora is less caring. "It's very important to me to be a good person," she has said. "If I die five years from now—and I have a one-in-five chance of being dead five years from now—I don't want to feel regrets. I want to live my life so that when I die, I'll know I did the best I could."

When she was first diagnosed, a friend and breast cancer survivor told her that she would get something out of the experience of having breast cancer. Nora responded, "Like fuck I will."

But when she looked back on the conversation, Nora realized that she was wrong. Having breast cancer *did* change her perspective. At two years after diagnosis, she feels that she has gotten rid of the "bullshit" of the film world. She found her friends to be overly caught up in "scenes": art scenes, film scenes. They placed more emphasis on being fashionable, on going to the right parties, and on knowing the right people, than she is now comfortable with. Having had breast cancer showed Nora that some of her pals were more "beer buddies" than close friends.

"Do you think you gained anything from having had breast cancer?" Mark once asked.

"I'll let you know in ten years," she told him, realizing that her perspective had changed. "If it doesn't kill me, then yes, I'd say I wouldn't trade the diagnosis for the world—for what I've learned." And she's not going to let it stop her. "If my time is up in five years, so be it. But I want to make sure that those next five years are completely over the top." And if that means asking for help again, so be it, she decided.

Nora went back to freelancing but, needless to say, she made sure she always had health insurance. "It's expensive, but it's *definitely* worth it," she told her mother, who breathed a sigh of relief.

Nora is still living in New York and has returned to working in television, though she now focuses on documentaries. She travels extensively for her work and has been to Jerusalem and all over Europe. Nora's health is good, and she has health insurance now. Dorian Gray, her cat, died one year after her mastectomy.

□ □ □

Lack of health insurance can be an enormous challenge for women diagnosed with breast cancer. Becky had no insurance when she was diagnosed and was only able to obtain barely adequate coverage after delaying definitive diagnosis and treatment for a month. The insurance company pointed her toward specific doctors, who did not fully meet her needs, which left her with huge bills that she was unable to cover even after she received payment from Supplemental Social

Income. Before Susan lost her job altogether, she worried about her company's decision to eliminate short-term disability insurance.

Insurance can be an issue for married women as well. While Paulette was able to switch jobs during treatment and after, she has sometimes relied on health insurance through her husband's employer. As a result, he has elected not to start his own consulting firm, so that he can maintain his insurance. Paulette and her husband worry that insurance companies will be hesitant to cover a woman who has had two mastectomies.

HMOs can also present obstacles at times. Paulette, for instance, had to delay starting chemotherapy treatment for two weeks to make sure she received appropriate treatment within her "network" to have it covered.

Young, healthy women often take insurance for granted, both medical and disability insurance. But women who have had breast cancer do not always have that luxury.

✧

Having breast cancer often spurs women to live life to its fullest. Once women are bluntly confronted with their own mortality, they are typically loath to waste time. And women who are still developing their careers, women forty and under, often use these insights to make changes in their work lives.

Some women, such as Anne and Nora, determine that their careers are immensely satisfying; others, like Janis, realize that their jobs are fulfilling but that their work/life priorities have shifted; and some find that their chosen careers are no longer meaningful, as Helen did. And they all want to have medical and disability insurance, just in case.

While specific career decisions vary, one point is consistent across these stories: Women who have had breast cancer don't want to waste their time. They want work that is interesting and rewarding. And they carefully balance that work with the rest of their lives. Living life to its fullest can mean having an exciting career—and it can also mean spending lots of time with family and friends. Every woman makes her own choice, but often, after breast cancer, survivors makes a more conscious decision.

Survivor Suggestions on Work and Career

☐ Work can help you cope with cancer treatment. Sometimes it can fill the time you need and give you a sense of identity. But don't let it overwhelm you and keep you from focusing on treatment.

☐ If you think continuing to work will help, talk to your employer about how to best combine treatment and work.

☐ If it is possible, don't stay at a job that is unsupportive.

☐ Set limits at work during treatment and after. Consider taking off nights and weekends.

☐ Be careful who you tell about your diagnosis—and how—in both social and professional settings.

☐ Be aware that government assistance might be available—and even necessary—to pay for medical treatment.

☐ Sometimes a lateral career move is the right decision for the family.

☐ Many women become politically and socially active after breast cancer treatment.

☐ Don't let breast cancer keep you from pursuing your dreams, professionally and otherwise.

꧁ Chapter Three ꧂

Sexuality and Dating

*How unfair, Mary joked, how unfair to have to worry about wigs
and scarves and still have to shave her legs.*

A BREAST IS NOT QUITE THE SAME as an ear or a toe. Breasts carry tremendous symbolic value; they remind us of our sexuality and of motherhood, they distinguish us from little girls and from men. It is no surprise, then, that having breast cancer often profoundly affects the way a woman views her body and her sexuality.

Most single women in their twenties and thirties spend at least some time dating and trying out new romantic relationships. The dating scene can be tough enough just as it is. Having breast cancer can really stymie dating in both physical and emotional ways. It changes a woman's sense of her body and sexuality—her feelings of self-worth, desirability, and sensuality. Young women with breast cancer worry about being seen as unable to be a life partner for someone, and some women struggle with self-doubt over perhaps not being able to bear children.

Not only the disease itself, but the ensuing treatment can also hurt a woman's self-image. During treatment, a woman can find it very difficult to date. Pinpointing a time when she doesn't feel sick, burned, or exhausted is tricky, let alone finding the energy to get ready for a date and trying to feel sexy, desirable, and attractive. Amanda, for instance, felt mutilated by surgery, bloated and bald from chemo, and burned by radiation. It is difficult to feel attractive and lovable when such a private and sexual area feels so violated.

Some women find the physical "scenes" of dating difficult to tolerate: They find it hard to hang out in a bar or attend an event because they cannot drink alcohol or because they get tired so easily. Becky, for one, found she sometimes had to leave a restaurant even before she and her boyfriend were seated.

A woman who is uncomfortable with the changes that have taken place in her body may be reluctant to share that body with someone else. Although this is true for women of all ages who are diagnosed with breast cancer, it is particularly true for women in their twenties and thirties, who are often looking for a life partner or are just starting to form stronger emotional and physical attachments. Becky, for instance, felt fragile and vulnerable during treatment. She was less willing to trust, more afraid of committing to a long-term relationship. But she came to terms with her fears and got to know a man during treatment, started dating him once she was finished, and married him two years after her initial diagnosis.

Coming to terms with a new, often different, body is a big part of dealing with the challenge of breast cancer. A flat chest resulting from mastectomy may become a constant reminder of something missing. So breast reconstruction helps many women feel better about their bodies. Amanda, for instance, worried that her husband wouldn't want her with only one breast. Reconstruction became a critical part of reclaiming her sexuality and her life.

But not everyone feels that way. Some women worry about the medical side effects of reconstruction. They see a mastectomy scar as a badge of honor, physical proof of their strength in overcoming tremendous adversity. For Mary, the scar itself instills confidence and pride. Nor has it stood in the way of her dating life; she is now married to a man she met after treatment, a man who respects her decision not to reconstruct her breast.

DATING? YOU'VE GOT TO BE KIDDING!

꙳᠌ Becky, 26: Wedding under the Arches

BECKY SAID "I DO" STANDING under the sixty-five-foot-high sandstone Delicate Arch in Utah's Arches National Park, overlooking a panoramic canyon view. She and Joshua* held hands while the mayor of Castle Valley officiated and about two dozen hikers served as witnesses. Becky swept back her now-wavy, shoulder-length hair and remembered herself two years earlier, when she looked like an ostrich, balding and too skinny from chemo; she remembered thinking she would never be healthy or happy again.

Then she looked over at Joshua, who had always seen her as beautiful, who helped her through diagnosis and treatment in a thousand little ways, and who brought her here to hike up mountains, rappel down canyons, and enjoy the most spectacular views imaginable. She never would have attempted such physical feats without Joshua's encouragement and example. For Becky, dating had been impossible during treatment and difficult afterward, but it was worth it.

The Red-Bearded Client
Becky was a dancer in New York City, with a typically busy dancer's schedule. In addition to dance classes and practices, she also taught dance and exercise and saw clients for personal training.

She started seeing her clients at six-thirty or seven o'clock in the morning. She met them at gyms around Manhattan or in their apartments to focus on stretching and strength building or in Central Park for power walks. She got along well with most clients, for whom she

*Not his real name

was as much cheerleader and taskmaster as exercise specialist. She particularly liked one client, Joshua, a muscular man with red hair, beard, and moustache.

After her early-morning clients, Becky typically took a morning dance class, then spent a few hours at the pottery studio, where she worked at a pottery wheel and threw pots, vases, dishes, and bowls. She often spent a few hours a day in dance rehearsals and taught five or six Pilates classes every week. She saw her personal training clients in the evenings, when she wasn't teaching aerobics at a local university. On a typical day, Becky wouldn't get back to her apartment in Queens until nine or ten at night. In between, she kept up with her friends and dated occasionally, though she was too busy for an intense relationship. Becky loved her varied days and depended on a date book to keep her straight.

Between her long hours and her intense exercise schedule, Becky was often tired. But so were all her dancer friends. Soon after she turned twenty-six, however, Becky started getting more tired than everyone else.

"Probably Just a Cyst"

One evening, when she couldn't sleep, Becky started dancing around her apartment wearing a camisole. Her straight hair hung midway down her back and swayed as she flitted around the room. As she drifted past the mirror, she caught, out of the corner of her eye, a strange shadow, a shadow she hadn't noticed before, on her left side, halfway between her nipple and her shoulder. Wow, she thought, that's not good.

Becky knew it was strange to see a lump in your breast. It's bad enough to *feel* it, she thought; she had never heard of anyone who'd found a lump in her breast by *seeing* it.

Becky didn't have health insurance, a gynecologist, or even an internist she saw regularly. It wasn't going to be easy to check the lump out. She called a few friends, got a referral, and set an appointment. Due to a change in scheduling, she ended up seeing a different doctor than the one for whom she had the referral.

"You're so young," said the doctor, who had been a dancer herself. "Given your age and the painful swelling you've been experiencing around the time of your periods, it's probably just a cyst."

"But my mother died three years ago of breast cancer, at fifty-one. She'd been in remission for seven or eight years; she was first diagnosed when she was forty-one. Isn't that something to worry about?"

"But you're so young," reiterated the doctor. "It's probably just a cyst."

Becky decided to see another doctor. She still had no health insurance, but discovered that dancers could purchase insurance through the Dance Theater Workshop of New York, though it would be expensive and would take a month to kick in. She decided to wait to see the second doctor because she worried that her insurance might not pay to treat a "preexisting condition" if anything was discovered before she was covered.

By the time she went back to her original gynecologist, the lump was bigger and felt like a small marble. But still, even with her family history, Becky had to convince the doctor to test her for cancer. Finally, the doctor relented and gave Becky a list of breast surgeons she had worked with.

Biopsy, Surgery, and a Welcome Visitor

The breast surgeon took one look at Becky and told her she needed to have her breast biopsied in the next day or two. "This looks serious," he said. "I wouldn't be surprised if there was node involvement." Becky made an appointment, canceled her classes and clients for the next two days, and went home to cry.

Fortunately, Becky was not alone on the day of her biopsy. She had told a couple of people, including her best friend, Andrea, and her sister, Jeanie, who lived in Boston, and happened to be in town for business. Technicians did a core biopsy, which was painful and very stressful for Becky.

Nearly two weeks went by before Becky learned the pathology results, which were positive for breast cancer. She was told she was a good candidate for a lumpectomy, followed by chemotherapy. Surgery to remove the lump was scheduled for three weeks later.

In one of the more disappointing non-medical developments, Becky was fired from several teaching jobs. "We just can't keep you on anymore," said her supervisor.

Becky called many of her clients and told them what was going on. Each one expressed concern, and Becky's apartment was soon overflowing with flowers. Joshua seemed particularly worried and called periodically to check up on her.

Becky was touched that so many people came to her surgery. Her father and stepmother came up from North Carolina and Jeanie flew down again from Boston. In addition, several local friends came, including Joshua, her red-haired client.

The breast surgeon excised Becky's tumor, leaving clean margins. After the surgery, Becky found she couldn't talk. She could hardly function; she felt like a zombie. Her friends and family entered her hospital room later on, looked worriedly at Becky, and cried—all of them.

"Becky, you look so tiny," said Joshua.

"I know," she sighed. "I look so sick." She didn't mention the scar, which started an inch below her collarbone. But she knew that very few shirts would hide it completely.

"No, you just look a little vulnerable. But you're still beautiful," said Joshua. "I wish there was a way I could help you."

"It's very kind of you to come visit," said Becky, who was a little embarrassed to have a client call her beautiful.

"I wanted to see how you are doing," said Joshua. "I know what I can do to help. My mother had breast cancer. She's a therapist and social worker and is very involved with breast cancer survivors. If I hook the two of you up, maybe she can give you some advice."

"Sure. I could use some help," Becky smiled.

⁂

Advice from a fellow dancer led Becky to explore Ki treatments, an alternative energy therapy. Two or three times a week, she saw a woman, Hiroko, who was apprenticed to a Ki master. Hiroko helped Becky with breathing techniques and visualization to channel her energy and help restore her depleted stock of energy. When Becky had the money, once or twice a month, she would see the Ki master. Sometimes, she would get Ki towels—regular paper towels that had been infused with Ki energy—and wear them under her shirt, against the scar.

"I know you don't understand," she told her family. "But I find this very mystical and powerful; it makes a big difference."

Bald Is Beautiful

Choosing an oncologist wasn't easy. On the recommendation of her surgeon, Becky initially saw an oncologist who treated mostly older, male patients. He wasn't able to tell her much about bone density loss, future fertility, or even the process of returning to daily living. Most of his patients had a spouse to help them or were financially able to hire a nurse.

Becky switched to another oncologist, who treated mostly young women. This doctor understood Becky's questions, knew the latest research on young women with breast cancer, and provided useful advice on nearly every question Becky posed.

Soon after, Joshua took Becky to meet his mother, Sara. Kind as Joshua was, Becky was embarrassed to need so much help; this didn't seem like the time to be making more attachments.

Sara was a therapist who'd had breast cancer herself, more than a decade earlier. She connected Becky with several organizations that could help her with medical questions and provide a hotline and a support group. As a result, Becky received one-time financial assistance that paid her rent for two months and bought some groceries. She also received some wigs, but they weren't quite her style—they were older women's styles and had gray hair. Possibly most important, the hotline and support group helped Becky feel less alone.

Before she started chemo, Becky applied for SSI disability benefits through the Social Security Administration to help pay her medical bills. There was a five-month backlog to have her application reviewed, then a three-month wait for a decision. So she crossed her fingers as the bills piled up. Becky received her first chemotherapy treatment in December and cut her hair short in anticipation of losing it. She was terrified of the experience, but had lots of friends and family supporting her.

The doctors installed an infusaport to deliver the chemotherapy just under Becky's collarbone. Becky was very uncomfortable having something foreign lodged in her skin. The medical staff told her she would have the infusaport throughout chemo and for several months to a year following treatment, in case the cancer should recur. That way, if there was another diagnosis, it would be easy to begin treatment immediately.

Joshua e-mailed every few days and brought her groceries and Chinese take-out. She was beginning to accept that he was more than just a client, though she wasn't quite ready to call him a friend yet.

෫℃ﭏ

After a few treatments, Becky lost all her hair. She had been terrified of being bald, but when she actually saw herself in the mirror, she loved it. Bandannas looked silly and hats felt wrong, so she just went bare-headed. Having no hair gave Becky a sense of freedom greater than she had ever felt before. And she felt beautiful—she'd never imagined how pretty her naked head would be. She felt modern and trendy and feminine and just gorgeous. She radiated beauty; her sister took photos, the women in the support group were envious of her obvious sense of liberation, and Joshua continually complimented her. But then she lost her eyelashes and didn't feel quite as attractive.

Feeling Unattractive

After three months of one chemotherapy regimen, Becky's doctors switched her to another chemotherapy cocktail. While the doctor was administering the first dose, Becky had a frightening allergic reaction, so they switched her to another medicine, a close cousin of the original drug. As a standard procedure, Becky started taking steroid pills before and after treatment to combat the side effects. The combination of steroids and chemotherapy wreaked havoc on Becky's personality. The steroids made her hyperactive and she was often awake and active for twenty hours at a stretch. Every two weeks, she received chemotherapy, which caused such fatigue and bone pain that she took four naps a day for about a week after the treatment. Shifting between hyperactivity and extreme fatigue was confusing, to say the least.

In addition, the steroids changed Becky's body. Not only did she gain back the weight she'd lost after surgery, but she put on an extra fifteen pounds and couldn't fit into her clothing. She had trouble adjusting to her rounder thighs and calves and her new size. In addition, her skin was pasty and her face had become wider.

These changes were depressing and made her feel unattractive. She felt so ugly she couldn't imagine dating. She didn't see how she could appeal to anyone and, in a way, she was relieved that she didn't have to worry about trying to hide her skin tone, stomach, and "moon face." She didn't think she would want anyone to touch her, so it was a relief not to have to think about it. She and Joshua had grown to become good friends by this time. But much as he said otherwise, Becky knew that he couldn't possibly find her pretty.

After her fifth chemotherapy treatment, Becky asked out-of-towners to stop coming by. She appreciated the help, but was becoming uncomfortable with being so dependent. It seemed like her tiny two-bedroom walk-up was getting smaller and smaller. She didn't feel very hospitable and wasn't up to making an extra effort.

Becky felt as though she had lost her independence. Daily life became a physical challenge. She could just about handle grocery shopping, but then it seemed almost impossible to carry the bags up one flight of stairs to her apartment. Often, she had food delivered. When they left it at the front door, the woman who lived downstairs would bring it up. When she ran out of clean clothing, either Andrea or her next-door neighbor would drop off and pick up laundry from the laundromat five blocks away.

Becky's finances were as much of a wreck as her body. Social Security rejected her request for financial support. Joshua was aware of her financial situation and offered to help her appeal to Social Security.

Through Joshua's father's law firm, they found a lawyer to help her and hoped for the best.

Three weeks after she finished chemotherapy, Becky started radiation, which she found degrading and disliked more than any other part of treatment. Appointments never started on time; she often had to wait as much as two hours. And she didn't like the way the radiology technicians treated her body. Ordinarily, she was very comfortable with her body and with being naked; she had posed nude for art classes and even danced without clothing. But lying naked on the table, being told not to move or breathe, and having technicians write on her with a ballpoint pen and markers made her feel like an object, not a person. "I felt like a science project," she told Joshua. The technicians put on some music, to try to take her mind off her body.

Trusting Her Body

Joshua, meantime, was trying to take Becky's mind off treatment and took her to a Rangers hockey game and a baseball game in the Mets-versus-Yankees "Subway Series" championship. He continued to shower Becky with kindness and compliments. It dawned on Becky that he was becoming more than a friend.

Becky really wanted to finish treatment and have her infusaport removed before she turned twenty-seven. And she did so, with thirteen days to spare. Joshua sent Becky a teddy bear on the day her port was removed.

✿

Becky's hair came back with a bit of "chemo curl" initially. After a few months, it grew in straighter, though with more wave than before. She liked her new look; she had always thought her hair was a little *too* straight. Once she was off steroids, she lost some of the weight she had gained and started feeling attractive again.

Around this time, Becky heard from Social Security. They had accepted her claim and sent her retroactive payment. But it still wasn't enough to cover all of her accumulated medical bills. Eventually and reluctantly, she accepted Joshua's assistance.

Once Becky was officially done with treatment, she was willing to start thinking about dating. Joshua sensed this and got a pair of tickets to a Keith Jarrett concert at Carnegie Hall. Despite all the times they'd been out together before, this time it felt like a romantic "date."

Becky was starting to fall in love with him, much as the thought scared her. She felt she had lost so much of her independence already that becoming emotionally dependent upon Joshua worried her. One weekend, when he returned from being out of town for a few days, Becky was livid. "How dare you make me miss you?" she exclaimed. He just laughed good-naturedly.

Hot Flashes on a Hot Date

Dating Joshua was sometimes difficult physically. On a dinner date, Becky would be exhausted before dessert. Or they would have such a long wait for a table that they would have to take a cab home before they were even seated. Joshua became very good at intuiting her needs. He could tell, often before Becky herself, when she could walk a block or two to the subway, when she was barely up to a bus ride, and when they would need a taxi.

Becky started taking tamoxifen after she finished treatment, which almost brought her back to her chemo state. She had hot flashes, mood swings, and weight gains. The hot flashes really interfered with their love life; often, when they kissed, Becky would get a flash and feel sweaty, uncomfortable, and unromantic.

Becky worried that Joshua didn't really understand what he was getting himself into. Did he realize that the cancer could come back, that she could die at any time like her mother had? Did he understand about children?

"I may not be able to have kids," she told him. "Even if I still have enough eggs after chemo, I'm not sure it's a good idea to get pregnant and increase my estrogen level that much."

"I know," said Joshua, who had attended plenty of doctor visits with Becky and was well aware of her medical condition.

"If you want to be with me, you need to do some soul-searching," she continued. "You need to be sure you would be comfortable with adoption."

Romance and Spinal Taps

"So, how long are we going to do this?" Joshua asked one evening.

"Do what?" said Becky.

"Dating. When are you going to move in with me?"

Becky changed the subject, not ready to think about becoming even more dependent on Joshua, much as she loved him.

After they had been dating for a few months, Becky started to have pains in her left arm. Her oncologist sent her to a neurologist, who was concerned about the possibility of metastasis and ordered a spinal tap. Although Becky's gut was telling her she was fine, she was still worried. Joshua went with her. Becky knew he hated needles, but she couldn't deny that she wanted him with her. She was scared. The spinal tap came back negative. But the doctor told her she would need two more spinal taps, just to be sure. They waited several days between them, to let her recuperate. After each one, Joshua took Becky home, stayed with her, and made sure she had plenty of food and water within easy reach.

The spinal taps were all decisive. Not only did they tell Becky that she had no new cancer, but they also proved Joshua's loyalty. "Anyone who could watch them do three spinal taps to me is really someone I can trust," she said told Joshua, and agreed to move in with him.

As Becky's energy increased, she would head out to Fairway, a large fruit and vegetable market in the neighborhood, for dinner fixings. It would take her an hour and a half to go the three blocks back to Joshua's apartment. She would lay everything out on the counter and start chopping scallions and other vegetables. Then she would sit down on the sofa to rest, just for a minute. A few hours later, Joshua would come home to a snoring woman and a counter full of minced vegetables.

"How long are we going to do this?" Joshua asked again one night as they started dinner with one of Becky's hard-won salads.

"Do what?" said Becky, though she thought she knew what he was talking about this time.

"Living together. When are we going to get married?"

"I don't know," said Becky in a sad voice. "I just don't think I'm ready for that."

Relearning To Dance

After almost a year away from dance, Becky found that she had a different body than she'd had before cancer. While still slender, she no longer fit the typical willowy dancer stereotype. She worried that her slightly more rounded appearance would affect whether choreographers would want to work with her. She had to remind her body how to move to music. She took the opportunity to teach it how to dance correctly, not just the way she had always moved. Having to relearn the dance movements made her a stronger dancer, she felt. "I move better, with more poise and confidence." Her strength and endurance had not yet returned to where they were before treatment: She couldn't lift her legs as high and her left arm wasn't as graceful as it had been. But at the same time, she had greater confidence in her ability to communicate through movement. "Dance is all about communicating and if I'm communicating better, then I gained something from all this."

Becky was also feeling good about her pottery again. She had been throwing pots all along, but her arm strength was compromised, and her weakness showed in her pottery. But now her work was slowly beginning to increase in size and skill. And people were starting to take notice; sales of her flowerpots and teapots were growing.

Joshua continued to broach the subject of marriage. In discussions with her counselor, Becky talked about her fear of losing her independence and her concerns about commitment. She mentioned how scared she was, given her mother's death and her own experience with breast cancer, how aware she was of her own mortality. "How can I get married when I could die at any time?" she asked.

When she spoke that feeling out loud, Becky had an epiphany. She realized that this feeling was always the case: Everyone is going to die someday. So why not get married to a wonderful man and be happy in the meantime?

She also told the counselor about her concerns over Joshua. Why would such a kind, generous man want to spend his life with someone who was so tired, so cranky, so frail? She didn't want to be responsible for ruining his life.

Once again, she told Joshua that she wasn't ready.

The next day, Becky splurged on a huge wedding magazine to look at the dresses and yearn. She had thought it would cheer her up to look at such beautiful pictures of such happy people, but instead the flamboyant photos were upsetting. She started to cry, thinking about the money she wasted on the magazine, moaning that she had told Joshua "no" and that now he would never want to marry her. When Joshua got home and saw her red nose and puffy eyes, she told him what she was feeling. He laughed, telling her it was the funniest thing he'd ever heard. "Of course I still want you," he said. "Why wouldn't I?"

Seven Blessings

When Becky and Joshua returned from their Utah honeymoon, they had a second, larger wedding, in New York's Fort Tryon Park, overlooking the Hudson River. The ceremony would be followed by dinner and a night of Cuban dance music.

This wedding represented a compromise. Joshua had wanted a small, private ceremony for just the two of them. Becky wanted a more public, family celebration. The legal proceeding had already taken place in Utah, so by the time they reached Fort Tryon Park, they could relax. They were already married and had taken their honeymoon.

The New York ceremony was a nod to Becky and Joshua's Jewish heritage. It included the seven blessings, which were made by relatives and her friend Andrea, as well as an impromptu eighth blessing provided by Becky's maternal grandmother.

At the end of the ceremony, Joshua stepped on the glass, a Jewish tradition that symbolizes the destruction of the Second Temple of Jerusalem and the comingling of sorrow and joy. For Becky, it was an apt reminder of the challenges of breast cancer and the pleasure and excitement of marriage. Even during such a difficult time, she found a man with whom to spend the rest of her life.

Becky and Joshua are happily married and living in Manhattan. Becky is now three years out from the end of her treatments, and will continue taking tamoxifen for two more years. She has some residual nerve damage to her left arm, and some lymphedema, as a result of her surgery, but otherwise is doing well.

□ □ □

Another common issue women face in the dating scene is that of disclosure and discovery. How much should they tell right away, how much should they share later on, how much is simply private and personal? Dana, going on one of her first dates with a new boyfriend, struggled over whether to hide her bald head or flaunt it.

Anne, who no longer has telltale signs when fully clothed, has decided not to date or even flirt for the time being; a man would see her scars before she would feel she knew him well enough to share her story. After breaking up with her first boyfriend post–breast cancer, she worried that men wouldn't be straight with her. She worried that they would break up with her, but not tell her the real reason. After her second cancer diagnosis, she was even more afraid to date.

"The problem with breast cancer and relationships is that things move more quickly physically than they do emotionally," she said. "I'm forced to tell someone pretty soon about the breast cancer. I have one breast with scars from a reduction and a silicone breast with a reconstructed nipple and a huge scar. It feels different than a natural breast. My second diagnosis makes it even more complicated. I suppose I could tell a man I started dating that I had breast cancer four years ago and not say anything about my current state. But what if we develop a relationship, and then three months later I say something about what's going on now. He would feel as though I hadn't shared. And if I do say up front, 'I have cancer in my bones and in my lungs,'—well, that's scary to anyone. I don't know if I can take the rejection now."

Once a woman discloses her medical history, it's hard to know how people will react. Anne's boyfriend just stopped calling after she told him what had happened. Similarly, Nora's boyfriend broke up with her while she was in treatment because, as he explained, *he* wanted to be the one to determine when the relationship would end; he couldn't handle the possibility of her dying.

But the flip side is true as well. Becky, Roberta, and Dana all dated during treatment and heard wonderful and supportive responses from the men they were seeing. All three of them found men so kind and caring that they married them. A partner who is understanding and compassionate can simultaneously provide tremendous support and prove him- or herself in ways that far outweigh mere words. Lanita, Helen, Janis, Barbara, and Dawn believe they never would have made it through their illness without the love and support of their partners. They found a renewed sense of being loved purely for being themselves, not for how they looked. In the long run, having breast cancer reinforced and strengthened their partnerships, it did not weaken them. Someone who can be there for you emotionally and physically when times are challenging, they suggest, will also be there during the trials and joys that constitute life after breast cancer.

HOW DOES BREAST CANCER AFFECT SEXUALITY?

🌸 Amanda, 35: Healing Arts

LOSING A BREAST, for Amanda, meant the diminution of her sexuality, her femininity, her nurturing ability, her womanhood. She wondered if her husband would still want her without a breast, or with an artificial one. And it just didn't seem fair.

After all, Amanda had always played by the rules. She went straight through from high school to college to a master's degree in health care management, she was a stable employee who rarely switched jobs, and she always made sure she had medical insurance. Even when Amanda took a new position because of an impending layoff, she planned ahead and had her annual physical right before the one-month insurance lapse. The doctor checked her slender, five-foot-seven frame from top to bottom, including doing a manual breast examination. Everything was fine.

But the very next month, February 1996, things began to fall apart for newlyweds Amanda and John. John took a tumble while skiing and needed stitches. And Amanda found a lump in her breast. While acknowledging how ridiculous it seemed, she was certain that if she hadn't had that lapse in insurance, the lump wouldn't have appeared.

Amanda found the lump one afternoon, when she was driving back from a meeting in Boston to her new job in Portland, Maine. For no discernible reason, her right breast hurt. Amanda pushed her long brown hair behind her ear and felt around her right breast, keeping her right hand on the wheel and her eyes on the empty stretch of interstate. Her breasts had always felt lumpy to her, but this was clearly a marble-size growth. When Amanda got home, she raced to her bedroom, flopped down on the bed, and called to her husband. "What is this?" she asked, pulling up her shirt and indicating the spot. Immediately John became quiet and serious, as he often did when asked a medical question. John was an emergency-room doctor, accustomed to remaining calm during medical emergencies. He felt her breast with his fingertips.

"It's hard. Does it hurt?"

"Yes," Amanda whimpered, terrified.

"It's so palpable," he mused. "It's a cyst," John continued confidently. "It wasn't there two weeks ago when you had your exam. It's a cyst, nothing to worry about." Amanda stared at him, puzzled at his certainty. "When our health insurance kicks in, make an appointment. You can even go to a family practitioner and she can aspirate it. It's no big deal."

Normal Test Results

Amanda waited. The physician she saw, a well-respected family practitioner, examined her and had the same response as John: "It is painful, easy to grasp, probably a benign cyst." Then he tried to aspirate it. He inserted the needle into the lump, but it didn't collapse as cysts are supposed to.

"That doesn't mean anything," the doctor reassured Amanda. "We'll send what we got off to the pathology lab and I'll call you as soon as I get the results."

For the next three days, Amanda was frantic, awaiting the results of the test. She tried to focus on her job in health care management at a recently expanding HMO, but whenever she forgot about the lump, the pain in her breast reminded her. Finally, the doctor called with the results.

"The test came back normal," he told Amanda, who responded with a huge sigh. "I'll continue to watch it; there's always a chance that the pathology test isn't perfect. Call me in a few months."

By April, the lump hadn't gone away, but it seemed smaller and flatter to Amanda. With this information, the doctor proposed waiting one more month. When the lump was still there in May, four months after Amanda's discovery, she called the doctor and told him she wanted a second opinion. She made an appointment with a surgeon recommended by some nurse friends.

"Take a seat on the examining table," the surgeon said. Amanda was surprised that he didn't have her lie down, as all of the other doctors had. He examined her breast and said that it felt fine.

"But it feels funny underneath the lump," said Amanda.

"That's probably just normal tissue that's compressed because of the lump," the doctor said, trying to reassure her. "The pathology test was normal," he continued, as Amanda buttoned her shirt. "You should probably have the lump removed, but there's no urgency." Amanda told him her mother's sister died of breast cancer at age thirty-seven; the doctor dismissed the information. "It's not a close enough relationship to affect your chances," he explained; only a first-degree relationship, a mother or a sister, matters. He suggested Amanda make an appointment with his secretary on her way out.

She set a date for mid-August. Amanda told herself that she was neurotic for worrying so much, that she should enjoy the summer and leave the surgery for when the Maine weather began to cool off. But as the months wore on, she began to get nervous again. The lump continued to be painful and it seemed to be growing. So she called the surgeon's office and begged his secretary to move the date up. The only date available was July 19, the day after Amanda's thirty-fifth birthday.

A Somber Celebration

Amanda's mother and father drove up from Boston to be with her after her surgery and bring belated birthday presents. When Amanda woke up from the anesthesia, she asked the nurse about the pathology results. "You'll have to ask the doctor, we don't know yet," she responded, quickly leaving the room. An hour later, the surgeon came in to tell her she could go home. Again, she asked about the pathology results.

"We couldn't complete the pathology testing because the tissue was too soft," he responded in a somber voice. "Come to my office on Monday, at the end of the day, and I'll have the results for you." Amanda pursed her lips, trying to form a follow-up question. The doctor looked over at John and said, "You're going to come with her, aren't you?"

John nodded, avoiding Amanda's questioning eyes.

⁂

For Amanda, the weekend was an intensified version of the seesaw she'd been riding since the spring. The doctor was so somber; there must be something seriously wrong. She'd been told she was fine by several doctors over a period of six months; surely they weren't all wrong. The doctor had asked John to come to the appointment; that wasn't a good sign. But if the results had been really terrible, the doctor would have known right away.

Amanda and John stopped off en route to the appointment at the beach in Portland. As they slipped off their shoes and settled into their spot on the sand, Amanda watched a group of children running toward the ocean waves. Quietly, without attracting John's attention, Amanda let tears start to roll down her face as she thought to herself, "I'm going to be getting some really bad news in about an hour. And what I really want to be doing is having children, not just watching someone else's kids play on the beach."

"Not What We Like"

"This is not what we like to have happen," the surgeon began obliquely. "I don't like to have told someone it was nothing and then have it turn out to be a malignancy."

Amanda and John were silent. *Malignancy, malignancy.* Amanda repeated the word over and over in her mind. The surgeon gave them the name of a well-respected oncologist in Portland who did a lot of breast cancer work and urged them to get an appointment as soon as they could. Amanda and John left the office and walked to a nearby field. They sat down in the grass and spent half an hour just holding each other and crying.

They didn't say a word. Amanda began to think about what would happen to her body. She had always felt insecure about her body and thought her breasts were too small. And now she might lose one. She wondered whether John would still love her if she had only one breast. At the same time, she felt some anger toward John; if he'd been a little more like her, a little more neurotic, maybe a little more thorough, perhaps the cancer would have been picked up sooner.

She felt guilty. She wondered how to break the news to her mother; she felt like she'd failed everyone in her family by being diagnosed with cancer. How could she get sick and let everyone down? She'd just started a new job and wouldn't even take a day off to go to New

York for a long weekend and now she's sick and needs surgery. She was supposed to take care of everyone, she thought, and now she'd let everyone down. And she'd disappointed John, too. While he hugged her, she continued out loud, "If you want to divorce me, I wouldn't blame you." John didn't say a word; he just squeezed her a little harder.

"I've never done drugs, I rarely drink, I don't smoke, I've always been empathetic," Amanda continued her thoughts aloud. "I've played by the rules my whole life. Maybe I should start smoking?"

"Breast cancer doesn't follow the rules," John said quietly.

A Second Second Opinion

Amanda made an oncologist appointment for that Friday afternoon. In the meantime, she spoke to friends and family members, received a hothouse's worth of flowers, bought a few books, and did a lot of research on breast cancer.

When they arrived for the appointment, the nurse led her back to an examining room and began asking a series of questions. She pulled out a Polaroid camera and asked to take Amanda's picture. Amanda nodded, then leaned over to John and said, "That's so they can compare how I look now with when I look really horrible." But she wasn't laughing when she said it.

Then the oncologist walked in and introduced himself. "Amanda's tumor was very large," he explained. "Approximately five centimeters. And it was necrotic, which means that it grew so fast it outgrew its own blood supply." He explained that a necrotic tumor was not a good harbinger for the future and began to talk about the possibility of her needing a bone marrow transplant.

"But won't that make me infertile?" Amanda asked, remembering her reading.

"Yes, but your own life comes first," the oncologist responded.

Amanda tuned out of the conversation. She thought about how she wanted to have children. She remembered how many choices she had made along the way to delay that. She had concentrated on her career in her early twenties, rather than thinking about marriage. She had chosen a man who put off their wedding for several years. Now, married and in a stable job, she was finally at a point where she could have the family she'd always wanted. Amanda simply was not ready to write all that off. Once again, she needed a second opinion.

Amanda contacted a physician friend who recommended an oncologist in Boston. Within two weeks, she had a day's worth of appointments to meet with the oncologist, surgeon, and radiation oncologist. "They will evaluate you and give you their recommendations," said the secretary. "Bring your pathology slides, X-rays, CAT scan, bone scans, and other test results."

Amanda met with each doctor individually. She explained to the surgeon that she was not interested in reconstruction. "I don't want to cloud the issue of the cancer. I don't want to mask any future growth," she said nervously. The surgeon spent a long time trying to convince her otherwise; she ultimately agreed to meet with a plastic surgeon at a later date. The three doctors conferred, then met with Amanda in a small office. The oncologist did most of the talking. "You're certainly going to need aggressive treatment," the doctor began. "But to qualify for a bone marrow transplant at this hospital, you would need at least ten positive lymph nodes. I would recommend doing the surgery first. Then we can decide about a bone marrow transplant." It scared Amanda that these doctors also thought a bone marrow transplant might be necessary; however, she felt some of the tension in her shoulders loosen. She was much more comfortable with their more conservative plan to wait to decide about a transplant. They recommended a modified radical mastectomy, then four months of chemotherapy, and then possibly six weeks of radiation. That didn't sound like fun, but it was a plan she could live with. They might determine she didn't need a transplant, and she might still be able to have children after all.

᚜᚛

Now that Amanda had a medical team in sync with her attitudes, she was ready to forge ahead with treatment. She sought and found support within the cancer community. She connected with a support group and a social worker who spent a lot of time answering Amanda's questions. They discussed reconstruction and Amanda came to realize that she *did* want to look as "natural" as possible. She saw how reconstruction could help her regain her sense of sexuality and womanhood and that it was not a selfish or medically unwise approach.

As a result of these discussions, Amanda decided on immediate reconstruction. The surgeon used the latissimus dorsi muscle in her back along with a small implant to make the new breast. He strongly suggested that she wear a Miracle Bra to ensure proper placement of the implant during the healing process. After surgery, Amanda felt more intact than she had imagined she would, and was thrilled to have *something* there, other than just a scar.

Just a Wig

Amanda had hardly had a chance to begin to come to grips with her new body when she began chemotherapy treatment, just three weeks after her surgery. She decided to continue to receive treatment in the same Boston hospital where she had her surgery. They knew her medical history and could easily communicate with her surgeon. Amanda liked the idea of having all her doctors in one place, and her friends generously orchestrated a system to drive her down over the following four months for her eight chemotherapy treatments.

Before she began chemo, Amanda cut off her chocolate-brown ponytail. She figured she would lose the hair anyway, and this way, she would be able to keep the ponytail intact. She set her hair aside, not sure what she wanted to do with it, but certain she wanted to keep it.

Amanda and John went out for dinner to celebrate their first wedding anniversary. Amanda was extremely sensitive and unhappy. She told John, "My hair hurts. I know that it's going to fall out soon. This is our first anniversary and I can't believe this is happening to me." She was right; her hair fell out the next day. Her eyebrows and eyelashes were soon gone, too, and she had scars on her back and chest from the surgery and reconstruction.

During chemotherapy, Amanda was constantly aware of losing her hair. At checkout lines and at every other opportunity, Amanda made certain to mention, "I have good hair, actually. This is just a wig."

John was puzzled; he just couldn't understand how self-conscious Amanda was about her hair. She still looked beautiful to him. He joked with her: "No one can tell that's a wig."

"Yes, they can. I know I can spot a wig a mile away."

Therapies and Supports

Amanda had hoped that the chemotherapy would be the end of her treatment, but her physicians decided that she would need six weeks of radiation as well.

The plastic surgeon wanted to make a bump for her nipple before she had radiation. "If you do the nipple first, there's a better chance that it will heal well."

"That's a cosmetic procedure," argued the radiation oncologist. "Your life is more important." The oncologist won that round. Amanda was a little disappointed, but the oncologist's argument was compelling. Amanda's company transferred her down to its Boston office while she was in radiation treatment. Every day at lunchtime, Amanda drove over to the hospital for her treatment. The radiation oncologist used towels to shield her surrounding skin and concentrate the radiation on her breast. Still, by the end of the six weeks, at the end of February, she had second-degree burns on her chest.

In March, after she completed radiation treatment, the plastic surgeon gave Amanda a new nipple. A few weeks later, it became infected. As Amanda looked at the wound on her chest, all she could think was: Why couldn't this simple little procedure work? The failed nipple came to represent all that was uncertain about breast cancer diagnosis and treatment. Within a month, her chest healed, and two months later, the plastic surgeon reconstructed the nipple a second time. This time, it took, though the reconstructed nipple was tiny.

Amanda joined a support group and remained involved with it throughout treatment. The group met in Portland twice a month and often had speakers such as nutritionists, journaling experts, and other mainstream and alternative-medicine practitioners. Partly as a result of the alternative techniques she discovered through the support group, Amanda began seeking other approaches to healing. She did healing touch, took diet supplements, and tried meditation, relaxation, and yoga. Amanda found these treatments very relaxing and affirming to enhance and complement the traditional medical treatment she was receiving. She tried to do better at forgiving people, including herself. She tried not to think that she somehow inadvertently caused her breast cancer; that attitude wouldn't help her emotionally or physically. It was important to Amanda to enjoy these alternative healing activities for their own value, not because they might "cure" her. That approach could set her up for disappointment.

Feeling Vulnerable

Amanda spent a lot of time during treatment worrying about the rest of her family. Her mother had lost her sister to breast cancer and Amanda knew she was thinking, "I can't do this again." The natural order of things is that children bury their parents, not the other way around. Amanda tried to convince her mother that she would be fine and was in control. As a result, John was really the only person who saw her fears, heard her complaints, and witnessed the physical toll that treatment took on her.

John represented another challenge. His emergency-room work wasn't as mobile as her office job, so he had to stay in Maine to work while Amanda received treatment in Boston. She could see how hard it was for him to give her back to her family, to let her mother take care of her. John was pulled in other directions as well. His mother, who lived in North Carolina, had had lymphoma, a cancer of the lymph nodes, which had been in remission for more than five years.

But that September, while Amanda was in chemotherapy, she had a recurrence and was put on very intensive chemotherapy as well. John decided to fly down to North Carolina to see his mother.

"I feel like I'm being upstaged," Amanda told John. When she saw the look on his face, she amended her words. "I mean, this is horrible for her—I can't imagine facing cancer a second time. But it's not very good for me, either. I feel like I need 150 percent of your attention right now. Instead, you're leaving town." Then, realizing how that sounded, Amanda pulled herself out of her self-focused cloud, back to her self-appointed role as caretaker. "I know this must be difficult for you. The two most important women in your life are struggling to stay alive. And you don't know what to do."

John's mother lost that struggle in February, at the end of Amanda's treatment cycle. This, too, terrified Amanda. She wondered when her time would come, but John kept telling her, "You are not going to die."

In February 1997, Amanda finished with treatment. But that, too, left her with mixed emotions. There was joy—the minute hairs began to sprout on her head, Amanda donated her one wig and the hats she had acquired during treatment to the American Cancer Society. It was liberating to give them away. But she felt emotionally fragile. Every little ache or pain sent her into a frenzy. She also felt unfeminine and unattractive. She couldn't address her concerns with John. Or rather, she could, but she didn't trust his answers. He tried to reassure her, but she dismissed all of his attempts, certain he was just being polite or humoring her.

Most of all, she felt vulnerable. For months, she had been in the hands of an oncologist, a breast surgeon, a radiation specialist, and other health care professionals. They were working to fight the cancer. But now she was on her own. She had to trust that she was going to be okay. And that was difficult. Having cancer had caused Amanda to lose her sense of security. She didn't look like the old Amanda and her body had betrayed her. At the same time, though, Amanda never lost sight of her main goal. She asked her doctor when she and John could try to have a child. Terrified as she was to trust her body, Amanda wanted to get on with her life. The doctors told her to wait a year.

About six months after she finished treatment, Amanda found she was less interested in going to her support group. Part of her really wanted to give back to the organization that had helped her handle her diagnosis and treatment. But part of her became outraged by the meetings; every time she went, there were two or three newly diagnosed women in attendance. Some were young women, a few even younger than she had been when she was diagnosed. She just wanted to go away, to avoid seeing that the breast cancer struggle was ongoing. Finally, she reached a balance, realizing that she could go only once every month or two. She tried to make sure that she felt good when she left the meetings, not upset, disturbed, or fearful.

In the summer of 1997, Amanda and John went to a dance concert at the Bates Dance Festival. They went every summer to see dancers from all over the country. Usually, Amanda focused on how gracefully the dancers moved, how lovely their bodies were. But this year, she just looked at the dancers' young, healthy bodies and envied them. She thought about the scars, the burns, and the mutilation of her body, the parts that were forever lost or changed in her fight against breast cancer.

"Now I Am Whole"

Art helped Amanda come to terms with her new body. Amanda went to an art workshop led by a local sculptor. Along with five other women in her support group, Amanda layered plaster-soaked gauze strips on her chest. Once the strips hardened to a breastplate, they were removed. After all the breastplates were dry, the group of women gathered and gazed in silence at the beauty of their changed bodies and shared their thoughts and feelings about the pieces. One woman suggested that Amanda's looked like a butterfly.

The next morning the women began to adorn their breastplates. Amanda remembered the earlier comment and decided to turn her breastplate into a butterfly. She used the ponytail that she cut off in the early days of chemotherapy, before she lost all her hair, as the body of the butterfly, laying it down in the middle of the breastplate with the unbraided end splaying at the bottom. She placed shells and a pearl on the right side, where her breast used to be.

"Making the casting was a way to reacquaint myself with my new body. It forced me to reconnect with myself," she told her friends in the support group. "The workshop helped me accept that my body is different and that I am different, but that that's okay. I am able to see myself as beautiful again."

Amanda named her breastplate "Metamorphosis" and wrote this poem to be displayed alongside it:

> I was diagnosed with breast cancer the day after my
>   thirty-fifth birthday.
> I had a modified radical mastectomy with immediate
>   reconstruction
> Followed by four months of chemotherapy and six weeks
>   of radiation.
> My hair fell out the day after my first wedding
>   anniversary.
> I sacrificed my right breast for my life.
> Now I struggle with the reality that my loss brings no
>   guarantees.
> I choose life. I am whole.

In August of 1999, after a miscarriage and an ectopic pregnancy, Amanda gave birth to healthy twin boys. She and John are still married and live in Maine. Amanda is eight years out from her diagnosis and is, as she puts it, "one of very few women who is happy to be over forty and getting wrinkled and gray."

⬜ ⬜ ⬜

Amanda is far from alone in worrying about her sexuality. Just about every story in this volume belongs here, as an example of coming to terms with changing sexuality. Some of the specific fears vary. Paulette knew her prosthesis didn't match her real breast; Roberta worried that she would never be able to change in a gym again; and Dana knew she wouldn't be herself until she could wear her bodysuit again.

But most of all, the survivors describe feeling unappealing and unattractive. Women who are dating wonder if anyone will ever want them, and married women worry that their husbands will no longer be interested. Despite repeated overtures, both Becky and Roberta maintained that their not-yet-boyfriends couldn't possibly be interested and were only being polite.

Many women continue to feel unattractive long after treatment is completed. Some continue to fight off weight gained during chemotherapy, others worry about the size and position of their scar. While she is still quite slender, Becky laments the loss of her dancer-lean body.

Feelings of sexuality are often, but not always, related to body image. Most women in this book felt uninterested in sex during treatment, both because they did not feel well and because they wanted to shield their bodies from even the most loving of eyes. But Nora's experience was quite the opposite; though she thought she was pale and overweight, she found that sex was the only time she felt alive during treatment. She and her boyfriend made love in places they probably wouldn't have considered under normal circumstances, including a cab at mid-afternoon.

While women's experiences and feelings of sexuality vary, one thing is certain: they have found ways to create a positive self-image from their newfound strength. They have created new visions of beauty and sexuality.

WHAT IF I DON'T WANT TO RECONSTRUCT?

✺ Mary, 36: Amazon Woman

MARY WAS PASSIONATE ABOUT BEING OUTDOORS. And while she was out there, she jogged or ran, skied or snowshoed, hiked or scaled mountains, or just went for a walk with a friend, preferably dressed in shorts and Birkenstocks. She didn't exercise just for exercise's sake. She never set out to tone her muscles or lose a few pounds—she felt very comfortable in her body—she just loved to be outdoors. And she loved living in Seattle, with its proximity to two large lakes and two major mountain ranges.

As an oncology nurse, Mary knew a lot about the physical and psychological effects of cancer. She'd been present for bone marrow transplants, stem cell transplants, and chemotherapy for more than a decade at one of Seattle's preeminent oncology wards. She'd administered chemo treatments and sat with patients to talk about how they were doing. In fact, that was the most meaningful part of her work: building long-term relationships with patients at a needy point in their lives. And as an outgrowth of her lifelong interest in alternative therapies, she was also pursuing a master's degree in acupuncture.

Because of her medical knowledge, Mary had always kept a close watch on her own body, carefully conducting breast self-exams every month. One morning, as Mary lay in bed checking her breast, she felt a firm spot. It had always felt firm just before she menstruated, but this time seemed different. It was a week before she was due for her period, so she decided just to keep an eye on the spot. She recalled the words of her family practitioner, "Your breasts have a graininess to them and you have various lumps that come and go. They're very hard to check. Chances are, you're the only one who will know if anything is wrong."

Mary's instincts were right. After her period was over, the firm spot was still there. And a week later, she could still feel it. Finally, Mary decided that it was time to see her new gynecologist. She called and got an appointment to see the nurse practitioner in two days. The nurse practitioner did an extremely thorough breast exam, assiduously checking and rechecking every bit of tissue. She agreed with Mary that there was something worrisome about the hard spot, and noted two other spots that warranted further investigation. Then she sent Mary down the hall to have a mammogram. The mammogram showed nothing out of the ordinary. But Mary remembered that this was often a problem with young women, especially slender ones like her; their breasts have so little fat that the mammogram reveals only dense tissue. The radiologist followed up with an ultrasound, which showed the culprit: a dark mass measuring approximately four centimeters. Then the radiologist performed a needle aspiration, all without so much as glancing at Mary's face.

A few days later, Mary got a call that the mass was "highly suspicious." In a daze, she made an appointment with the recommended breast surgeon. The breast surgeon recommended an incisional biopsy, rather than removing the entire large lump, so he could get enough tissue for definitive pathology results. As Mary came out of the anesthesia, still groggy and only half-awake, lying on the operating table, the surgeon said, "It's cancer." Then Mary drifted back into slumber. She woke up in the recovery room and began to cry. Through her tears, she tried to describe how she felt. "It's not that I'm scared," she began. "I'm just very sad." She gulped. "I know I'm not going to die, I know I'm going to be okay. This is just a journey that I need to go on and see what I can learn. But I'm really sad right now."

A Multi-pronged Approach

The first month after the diagnosis, Mary felt caught up in a whirlwind. Fortunately, she knew people in the medical community because of her nursing background. A physician friend gave her the names of five reputable oncologists, men and women, and Mary talked to them all. She questioned each doctor closely, checking out his or her interpretation of Mary's diagnosis and proposed methods of treatment, attitudes toward alternative medical treatments, and bedside manner. She realized it was going to be a long-term relationship. She wanted someone knowledgeable, but also someone she could talk to, someone who would listen to what she had to say.

Mary felt most comfortable with the last doctor she spoke with. They discussed possible treatment options and Mary's plan to use alternative means in addition to traditional Western methods. The doctor seemed very comfortable with a multi-pronged approach to cancer treatment.

Since the tumor measured approximately four centimeters on the sonogram, the doctor recommended a magnetic resonance imaging (MRI) test to determine the exact size. The test showed two hazy spots near the center of the breast. The oncologist wasn't sure exactly what those spots were, but he was concerned.

"You can either do chemotherapy first to help shrink the tumor and kill any cells that might have spread, and then have surgery," said the doctor. "Or you can start with surgery and then do chemo. To be honest, though, I'm a little concerned about those two gray spots, so I would recommend starting with chemotherapy." Mary nodded. She wasn't scared of chemotherapy, partly because she was familiar with the process. She trusted her body to mend itself and chose to view chemo as "healing juice."

With her boss's blessing, Mary took a leave of absence from her job at the clinic to focus on healing. Her colleagues from the clinic were equally supportive. Every Friday evening, someone from the clinic came over with piping hot soup or one of Mary's favorite organic sandwiches. Mary decided to finish her acupuncture degree despite her diagnosis. Her teachers and classmates were all supportive and willing to talk and take notes for her when she was unable to come to class. They even arranged to have her Eastern vitamin supplements donated for six months.

She kept up her health insurance, but had no income once she stopped working. Mary really wanted to be able to keep her own place, to feel independent at least in her daily activities, if not financially. Her parents paid her rent, and she used up her savings.

Cancer Camp

Mary's older sister, Lisa, moved in for the summer. A year and a half older than Mary, Lisa stood the same height as her sister but was much more fair, with blond hair and light-blue eyes. A CPA, she loved to experiment in the kitchen, do needlepoint, and check out garage sales. She'd had a baseline mammogram a few months earlier, near her home in Hawaii, which showed some calcifications in her left breast. Her doctors diagnosed hyperplasia and recommended that she be checked again in six months. Lisa came to Seattle for Mary's graduation from her acupuncture program. When she heard about Mary's diagnosis, she got nervous and decided to have her checkup in Seattle, with the doctors Mary had found and respected so much.

The Seattle doctors read Lisa's biopsy slides and mammogram differently than her Hawaii physicians had. They diagnosed ductal carcinoma in situ, a localized cancer.

"We had no family history until now," Mary noted. "But I guess we're starting one."

"I guess so! So, I'll just stay here with you and we can have Cancer Camp," Lisa joked.

Lisa opted for a wider excision of her biopsy, followed by radiation therapy for three months.

Mary and her sister quickly settled into a routine. Monday mornings, Mary went in for her chemotherapy treatments. Either her sister or her mother went with her, so she was never alone. Each week, the oncology nurse drew Mary's blood, ascertained whether her blood count was high enough for the week's chemo treatment, and administered the drugs. Mary saw her doctor, just to check in, then took it easy for the rest of the day.

Lisa had radiation treatment every weekday morning at about 8:30. Then the two sisters went for a three-mile walk around Green Lake, located a short distance from the apartment. Some days Mary walked quickly, other days she was sluggish. It was important to Mary to get outside, enjoy the fresh air, and get her body moving every day. After her walk, she lay down for a "healing interval," listened to affirmation and guided-imagery tapes, and took a nap. After her nap, the sisters typically went to their parents' home for dinner. Chemo made Mary mildly nauseated initially, and the anti-nausea drug made her feel even worse than the treatment. But once Mary settled on a combination of Chinese medicine, acupuncture, and a daily antacid, she had no more trouble with nausea. In fact, her family joked, "You eat like a horse."

About a month into chemotherapy, Mary could sense that she was going to lose her waist-long tresses and called her hairdresser, Anthony.

"My hair is starting to come out," she said. "My graduation is this weekend and I don't want to be totally bald. Could you cut it for me so that I still have some on my head, but also have enough to make a wig?" Anthony cut Mary's hair to a layered cut just above her ears, and gave her five ponytails in a clear plastic bag to take to the wig-maker. At her graduation, Mary was pleased to hear the many compliments on her new hairstyle. A week later, on Father's Day, the family gathered for a picnic with cousins, aunts, uncles, and friends of the family. But this wasn't just any family picnic: Her relatives had created a wig fund, donated money, and raised $1,000—exactly the price tag for the custom, real-hair wig Mary had in mind. With the family's check in hand, Mary gave the bag of ponytails to a company in the area, which wove a soft, natural-hair wig out of Anthony's clippings. It took three weeks to complete the project, but the result was well worth the time and expense. As Mary told her family, "If I want to wear hair during chemo, I want it to be *mine*." (But as it turned out, Mary found she was a hat-and-scarf girl during treatment.)

Lots of Hats

Breast cancer taught Mary how to ask for help. "It makes me teary-eyed just to think about the amount of love and support that is out there," she told Lisa as they traversed the lake on a balmy Saturday afternoon.

"You just have to respect how involved people want to get. Some people can't be in the thick of things; they might want to cook a meal or clean the house or give me a ride or go for a walk." Mary stopped to look out on the water, pointing out a speedboat rushing by. "Other people can go to chemo appointments or doctor's visits, or just talk when I'm feeling upset. Most people are more than happy to be supportive; it's just a matter of figuring out what they can do. And not being afraid to ask."

Mary's friends from acupuncture school threw her a head-shaving party. About a dozen friends came. "What a wonderful ritual," Mary said, "to acknowledge what's going on." That evening, though, Mary wasn't quite ready for a *total* shave.

"Just take it down to about an inch," she asked her friends as she handed over the buzzer. Mary sat on a chair on her front porch surrounded by her friends and relatives. She closed her eyes, squeezed her hands together nervously, and smiled. She felt the buzzer vibrate against her head and opened up her eyes to watch her hair fall on the wooden planks. When it was finished, a friend handed Mary a mirror. She took one look at the short pixie cut and sighed. "You should have been a hairdresser; this looks great!" As Mary stood up, she noticed a dozen beautifully wrapped boxes on the porch steps. Opening the boxes, she found a collection of baseball caps, flouncy cotton hats, berets, and straw hats.

The following weekend, as Mary was lathering her newly cropped hair, it came out in her hands. She gasped as she held a handful, and sat down on the toilet to stare at the remains of her light-brown hair. Then she stood up, washed the rest of the hair down the drain, and telephoned a friend to come shave the rest of it off. When her friend put down the buzzer, Mary took a look in the mirror. "This is very liberating!" she said. She had no hair on her head, hardly any eyelashes, and no pubic hair to speak of. All she had were her eyebrows and the hair on her legs. How unfair, she joked, how unfair to have to worry about wigs and scarves and to still have to shave her legs.

Going the Distance

During Mary's second month of chemotherapy, a nurse handed her a flyer about a triathlon. She said, "They're putting together a team and we thought of you."

"I don't think I'll be doing a triathlon any time soon," Mary laughed. Then she looked more closely at the flyer. The organizers of the triathlon were hoping to put together a team of breast cancer survivors and part of the competition proceeds would go to breast cancer research. "Maybe I could *walk* one of the events. Maybe I could even run that far." Then Mary noticed that the triathlon was in two weeks. That afternoon, Mary called the phone number on the flyer. Eight women had signed up for the team and Mary decided to join them. I'll just go out there, jog, and see how I feel, she thought. She ran five times before the race and got up to a mile and a half before she had to slow to a walk.

Race day was a sunny Sunday morning. Mary felt good as she hung her number card around her neck and sauntered over to the starting line. A woman she had never seen before approached her and asked, "Would you like me to run with you?"

"Sure," Mary replied, thinking that it was kind of the woman to offer, and that the encouragement would be helpful. They jogged the first mile and Mary thought about whether she should slow down. She decided to keep jogging. When they got to the second mile, farther than she had gotten during training, she kept on going. They ran the whole three miles together. Mary was no speed demon, but she was proud that she could keep a steady pace.

Mary wasn't the only team member who found the triathlon fun and invigorating. The women decided to continue to meet as an ongoing support and activity group for female cancer survivors. Over the next two years, the group grew to include about a hundred regulars of all ages, diagnoses, and types of cancer. Some women were newly diagnosed, others were mid-treatment, and one woman was twenty years past diagnosis. Like traditional support groups, this group provided the information exchange and psychological help that can make a big difference in recovery; in addition, the group motivated the women to live a healthy lifestyle. Activities ranged from hiking to cross-country skiing to snowshoeing. A few members, including Mary and Lisa, even climbed Mount Rainier. Mary also joined a traditional support group and attended meetings weekly. She found it useful to share information, advice, and psychological support with other survivors.

Getting Rid of the Gray Spots

After three months of chemotherapy, Mary's tumor had shrunk considerably—enough to consider a lumpectomy. The oncologist did an MRI to gauge the exact size, then gave Mary one more month of chemo. When the tumor didn't shrink any more, he decided it was time to operate. He gave her one more month to rest up and to get her blood cell counts back up.

At the end of September, when Mary was finishing up chemo, Lisa finished her own treatment and returned to Hawaii. "Don't worry," she promised. "I'll be back for my six-month checkup."

Mary's next step was surgery. Her doctor recommended a mastectomy because of the two gray spots on the MRI. Even though the spots disappeared after the chemotherapy treatment, he wasn't comfortable performing a lumpectomy. "I've really struggled with this one," he began. "But from a medical standpoint, I have to recommend a mastectomy."

Mary had hoped for a lumpectomy; she didn't want to lose her breast. She consulted with several other surgeons, all of whom told her the same thing: Play it safe, have a mastectomy just in case. She spent a lot of time thinking about this decision.

"I don't want to spend the rest of my life wondering what those two gray spots were," she told her sister. "Were they cancer? Or not? And most important, if they *were* cancer, are they *really* gone now? Or are they going to grow?"

Lisa was quiet.

"I guess I'll have a mastectomy," Mary said slowly. "I know it may be more than I need to do, but if I have my breast removed, I'll know that those gray spots are gone. I won't have to worry about leaving anything behind."

"And you won't have to have radiation," her sister added.

But Mary continued to struggle with the idea. She began doing more intensive visualization, listening to more relaxation tapes. One tape took her all the way from the moment she was at home packing her bags for the hospital through coming out in the recovery room. She listened to it nonstop for three days until she was able to view the mastectomy not as an attack on her body but as a way to heal.

Honor the Sacred Space

Mary decided to take a mini-vacation the week before surgery. A colleague offered her the use of a cabin on the Oregon coast and Mary took off with a friend. They spent the week flying kites, taking long walks on the beach, and watching major league baseball playoffs on TV. While she was there, Mary also attended a retreat for cancer patients in the area. She met a woman who had recently had a lumpectomy and had spoken with her surgeon moments before the surgery to explain how she felt. "I talked to him about how important my breast was to me and I asked him to honor it." That approach made a lot of sense to Mary.

When Mary got back to Seattle, she was feeling a little more prepared for surgery. The morning of the operation, she spoke with her surgeon, bearing in mind the words of the woman at the cancer retreat.

"I want to ask you to do something for me," she began as the surgeon listened attentively. "My breast is very important and I am feeling a little nervous about this surgery. Please honor my body and the sacred space you are going to be working in."

"I understand how you feel," the surgeon responded in a gentle voice. "My wife had breast cancer and I can appreciate how difficult this is for you." He paused, then added, "She's fine now." As he stood up to prepare for surgery, he mentioned one more detail. "The surgical nurse I'll be working with had breast cancer, too, about three years ago. You won't be alone in this. Don't worry."

Mary had a relatively calm night after the surgery. When she awoke, she lifted up her gown and stared at the clear dressing over her chest. The scar was longer than she had thought it would be, but certainly not as ugly as she had feared. "I can deal with that," she said to herself.

When the surgeon came to check up on her, Mary asked, "Can I do the Race for the Cure in four days? It's only three miles and I'm not going to run. But I do want to try to walk it."

"If it's not raining, I don't see why not," the surgeon responded with a smile, as if to say, the request didn't surprise him. "If it's raining, you should probably stay home because your [blood cell] counts are a little tenuous and we don't want you to get sick." Mary prayed for good weather.

Race day came in bright and sunny once again. Mary walked the race, along with her sister, her mother, and all the women from her activity support group.

Mary took a month off after surgery to give her body time to rest before resuming chemotherapy. None of her lymph nodes were positive, and she remembered how she had conquered the nausea, so she wasn't worried about the final two months of treatment. But she wasn't looking forward to them, either.

The first month was hard on Mary's body, harder than the first six months had been. Her combination of Chinese medicine, acupuncture, and antacids wasn't working this time. She was nauseated and so tired that some days she didn't even have the energy to zip up her jeans. Finally, she asked her oncologist for suggestions.

"You've been doing fine so far," he said. "Let's just drop one of the drugs for the last month. I think that will help." He was right. The day after she stopped taking the one drug, she felt fine.

Making Changes

When she finished chemotherapy, Mary noticed her focus shifting. It was as though now that she had finished her treatment, she could start thinking about life beyond chemo. Not that she hadn't been living up until then, and making short-term plans for dinners, triathlons, races, and other events. But now she could make plans for the future. She realized that being in treatment had taken all her focus and energy—concentrating on keeping up her routine, making medical choices, and enduring treatment had been her full-time job for months. Now that she didn't have cancer anymore, she could actually consider her long-term future.

One of the first choices she made was to start anew and to move south to Boulder, Colorado, a smaller city than Seattle. She wasn't running away from anything in particular, but just wanted a little more sun, a smaller city, and a location closer to the mountains. Most of all, she wanted a lower-key lifestyle, a place that moved at a slower pace and offered a little more elbow room. So, two years after completing treatment, she rented a car and drove all over Colorado, to get a feel for the state and decide if she wanted to live there.

She stayed with a friend who wanted to show her some photographs that were hanging in the lobby of a nearby clinic. The photos were of children going through chemotherapy; the kids were in action—riding their bikes, kicking balls, running around. While they were looking at the uplifting photographs, Mary recognized some names on the building directory.

"I know two of these doctors," she said. "I used to work with them in Seattle. I didn't know they'd moved down here. I'd like to go say hello."

They went up to see the physicians and tour the clinic, ending up in the director's office. The doctors whispered to the director, who then introduced herself. "Do you want a job?" the director asked. "Well, yes, sure," Mary responded with great excitement. Three weeks later, she moved into a beautiful apartment in Boulder and began working part-time as a nurse at the clinic.

Meeting Mr. Blue-Eyes

Not long after moving to Boulder, Mary met Andy in an outdoor-sports store. At six feet tall, with dark brown hair, a moustache, a goatee, and marine-blue eyes, he was striking. Despite her initial reservations—Mary wasn't sure she was ready to initiate a relationship so soon after fighting breast cancer and moving to Boulder—they began to date. Andy loved the outdoors as much as Mary, and together they biked, ran, and went cross-country skiing, rock climbing, and hiking. Within three weeks, they were engaged. Mary didn't expect things to move so quickly, but she had never met anyone who made her feel as comfortable as Andy.

Amazon Woman

Mary chose not to reconstruct her breast following her mastectomy, deciding to live with just one breast. "The biggest challenge has been to learn to trust myself after the mastectomy," she said. "I feel okay the way I am. I love my body and I have no trouble with pain or swelling in my arm, or range of motion, or any of the other problems that sometimes come along with reconstruction. I'm a very active person and I'm not willing to sacrifice the way my body works simply to have a second breast."

"Do you miss having two breasts?" asked a new member of her Boulder support group on their weekly jaunt around a lovely lake.

"There are definitely some days when I would love to have two breasts. On those days, mostly in the summer, I wear a prosthesis; I just Velcro it into my bra. When I go braless, it would be nice if I were symmetrical."

"Do you wear a bra?" the woman gasped; she hadn't been on this long a walk since before her own diagnosis.

"Some days I do, some days I don't."

"What does it feel like, to have only one breast swinging around?"

"It doesn't exactly swing." Mary laughed. "I'm pretty small-chested."

"What do you wear to go swimming?"

"I wear a jogging bra and my swimsuit bottoms."

"No prosthesis?"

"No," Mary laughed again. "I don't wear a prosthesis when I go swimming."

"But," the woman began, then paused, suddenly embarrassed by her forwardness. "Don't you worry about what people think?"

"I think the struggle is probably what is important to me, as opposed to what is important to society. My mom and dad love me, you love me, my fiancé loves me. The people who love me accept me the way I am. And I don't worry if there are people who wonder." Mary lifted up a branch that was hanging over onto the path. "I guess this is how I make people aware of breast cancer. People look at me and think, 'Well, she obviously had breast cancer and had her breast removed.' But then they see that I'm healthy, that I'm swimming or hiking or whatever. And I hope that increases their awareness of their own uneasiness and where it comes from. I like to think that it changes the face of cancer for them."

"It really just doesn't bother you?"

"Some days I wonder why I have to worry about it, other days I don't even think about it at all. I think maybe it's a test of my own fortitude, in some ways. And I may decide someday to have reconstruction, I don't know. But for right now, I'm okay with the way my body is." Mary paused. She plucked a big leaf off a tree and fanned herself for a moment, then dropped it onto the grass.

"It reminds me of Amazon women. In the legend of the Amazons, female warriors would cut off one of their breasts so that they could use their bows more efficiently and be better warriors. I think that's a nice way of looking at it," she said, straightening up. "Because, in a way, I think of myself as a breast cancer warrior, having survived a life-threatening disease. Having my breast removed, having the mastectomy, made me a better warrior, in a sense. It helped me win the war against cancer." Mary held out her hand and helped the woman sidestep a large hole in the path; the woman smiled.

Mary and Andy were married a year and a half after they met. They continue to live in Boulder. Mary works part-time as a nurse and is heavily involved with the activity support group Rocky Mountain Team Survivor. She is in good health.

□ □ □

Survivor Suggestions on Interacting with Friends

☐ Friends who treat you like you aren't sick are golden; let them do it.

☐ Accept help from family and friends.

☐ Take care of your support system; give them time and space to come to terms with the situation, the way they are doing for you.

☐ People want to be helpful; when keeping their distance would be useful, let them know. Understand the limits of family and friends; let them help in the way that they are most comfortable.

☐ Realize that some friends may disappoint you, but most won't. Figure out who you can count on for support, and who simply cannot be there for you. Don't focus on the friends and relatives who failed you; think about the ones who were really able to support you and help out.

Deciding whether to reconstruct is an enormous and very personal undertaking. There are medical, aesthetic, and sexual aspects to consider. For some women, it is a question of balance, of wearing clothes comfortably. Roberta, for instance, realized that not being lopsided would make it easier to dress and to regain a sense of balance. Dana knew that the day she could wear her bodysuit again, she would feel okay.

Others see reconstruction as a matter of completion, of becoming whole, of returning to "normal." Paulette saw the prosthesis and the flat part of her chest as unremitting signs that something was missing. Janis admits that she would have had a more difficult time with breast cancer if she had woken up from surgery to find only one breast.

For some women, having to have breast surgery and reconstruction is an opportunity to change their physique. Anne had a simultaneous reconstruction in one breast and reduction in the other. Lanita, who had a prophylactic double mastectomy, convinced her doctors to use the smallest size of implants available and to make them even smaller.

Reconstruction is not always a permanent solution to the issue of symmetry, however. Jacquie, for instance, at twenty years post-treatment, has gained weight and now finds that her natural breast is noticeably larger than her reconstructed one.

Mary, as we have seen, prefers the badge of honor that an unreconstructed breast symbolizes. As a very active woman, she wanted no possibility of side effects getting in her way. For her, asymmetry is a source of pride, not regret.

Whatever decision a woman makes about reconstruction, there are other young women who have made the same choice. And who feel good about it.

↭

Breast cancer leaves a woman's body in a different state than it was before diagnosis. Both the disease itself and its treatment lead to wear and tear on a woman's body and young women feel these changes acutely.

These women may be burned from radiation, bloated and balding from chemotherapy, and scarred from surgery. A woman may feel unattractive and unsexy, and worry that no one will ever want to look at—or touch—her body again. But as the stories in this chapter demonstrate, there are many ways women learn to reawaken their sexuality and to love their changed bodies. Breast reconstruction was critical for Amanda, and she came to closure with her breast cancer through the healing powers of art. A return to physical activity helped Mary and her sister. And love from a caring man allowed Becky to feel better about herself and her body.

Having breast cancer forces women to think anew about how they view themselves and their bodies, and about what they value in a relationship.

Survivor Suggestions on Sexuality and Dating

☐ Don't be afraid to date during or after treatment; someone who can love you when you are ill and bald is someone special and can probably handle other life challenges.

☐ Consider reconstructing your breast. It might help you feel better about your body. But don't feel you have to reconstruct; do what feels right for you.

☐ If you decide to reconstruct, use the opportunity presented by breast surgery to get the breasts you've always wanted, larger or smaller.

☐ Looking at the scar is not as bad as avoiding it.

☐ Bald can be beautiful.

☐ If you choose wigs, use them as a chance to be someone you've always wanted to be.

☐ Think of your body, including the site of the surgery, as "sacred space."

☐ Learn to trust your body during treatment and after.

☐ Find new ways to think about your sexuality.

☐ Believe it when your husband, boyfriend, or partner says you are attractive.

Chapter Four

Pregnancy, Children, and Family

Eighteen-month-old Claire pointed at
Paulette's chest and asked, "Where is it?"

IT'S HARD NOT TO BEGIN A SECTION ON THE JOYS of young motherhood with a series of clichés: the gurgle of gratitude that accompanies a particularly messy diaper change, the pleasures of cuddling and reading picture books, the jolt of satisfaction when you are beamed in the head by the first successful ball toss.

But it simply isn't true that having children makes a woman feel immortal. Instead, as Barbara Kingsolver has written, having little lives to watch over makes a woman feel, if anything, *more* vulnerable than ever. With children, a woman's life takes on more importance; she worries who will make sure the kids have peanut butter sandwiches and milk money if she isn't around.

Young women face questions about whether—and how—to have children. Jacquie, for instance, decided on adoption, realizing that childbirth wasn't an option anymore. Meanwhile Susan elected, at age forty, to become pregnant and raise her child as a single parent.

Mothers who are in breast cancer treatment, such as Barbara, confront logistical challenges. When you work first shift and your husband works third, who gets the kids off to school when you are ill from chemo?

Also, mothers have to figure out how to explain what is happening to their little ones. How do you tell a small child, as Paulette had to, that, "mommy isn't feeling 100 percent?" It's hard to explain the physical changes—the surgery, prosthesis, hair loss—taking place in your body. And, as Barbara found, it is difficult to help your children understand their heightened risk of breast cancer.

Some women must also tackle the question of genetics. In between her first and second mastectomies, Paulette found out she has the BRCA1 breast cancer gene. How can she explain this to her daughter, born before she found out about her genetic predisposition toward the disease? Should she have her daughter tested?

Parenting can be a challenge in and of itself. But when you add the physical and psychological issues of breast cancer to the mix, it may seem insurmountable. But at the same time—as Susan, Jacquie, Barbara, and Paulette attest—parenting is incredibly life-affirming. It is, as Susan says, what she wanted most in her second chance at life and it brought her—and Jacquie, Barbara, and Paulette—the greatest of joys.

WHAT IF I WANT TO HAVE CHILDREN?

Susan, 40: Breast-feeding in Dana Farber

THE ONCOLOGY NURSE LED SUSAN to a small room with a lavender overstuffed chair and a panoramic view of the Boston Harbor. Dana Farber Cancer Institute, one of the nation's premier cancer hospitals, was located right on the waterfront and the ninth-floor oncology ward offered particularly spectacular vistas. Eleven-week-old Diana fussed

*Not her real name

quietly while Susan put her purse and diaper bag at her feet, positioned the baby in her lap, and unhooked her nursing bra. Diana latched on immediately and began sucking voraciously.

As Diana's little body calmed itself and curled around her mother, Susan could feel herself relaxing as well. She knew that part of the peaceful feeling flowed from the endorphins her body released when the baby suckled. But most of her mood stemmed from the triumphant feeling of breast-feeding her infant daughter here, in the hospital where she received part of her treatment for breast cancer, where she had worried whether she would ever have children.

Susan had approached her fortieth birthday feeling depressed. She had realized that, more than anything else in the world, she wanted to be married and have children. And she was nowhere near reaching either goal. As she turned the page on her thirties, both goals had felt even more remote. The more she thought about her situation, the sadder she felt. She debated whether to see a psychiatrist for an antidepressant prescription. Then something happened to take her mind off children.

She was diagnosed with breast cancer.

※⊃෴

When Susan turned forty, she went in for her first "real" mammogram; they'd done a baseline at thirty-five and another at thirty-nine, but this was the first regularly scheduled mammogram. "There's something suspicious here," said Susan's gynecologist. "We need to take more films and do an ultrasound."

The additional tests pointed to a radial scar. "Some radial scars are benign," the doctor said, "but some are associated with cancer."

"What do you do now?" Susan asked, starting to worry.

"Due to the nature of radial scars, a needle biopsy wouldn't be conclusive. A positive result would be conclusive, but a negative result wouldn't necessarily rule out cancer. So we will need to do a surgical biopsy," the doctor explained.

"I'm too young to die," said Susan.

"You're going to have to find something else to die of," reassured the doctor. "You're not going to die of this."

Susan ended up having a needle biopsy preliminarily. The results were negative, so it was followed up by a surgical biopsy. The wide excision, or lumpectomy, was positive for cancer.

Susan's oncologist offered her the choice of mastectomy or lumpectomy with radiation. Because her diagnosis was nonaggressive ductal carcinoma in situ, or DCIS, with no node involvement, she was lucky and wouldn't need chemotherapy; as a result, her fertility was unlikely to be affected. Nevertheless, Susan was nervous about the treatment decision and asked her doctor, "Do you think I should have a mastectomy, just to be safe?"

"A lumpectomy, radiation, and careful observation are reasonable in your case," she responded. "But there are no guarantees."

Susan decided she liked having two breasts; it made her feel like a whole woman. They made her feel sexy and desirable. She hoped to marry one day and wondered what sexual intimacy would be like with only one breast. So she decided to have a lumpectomy, hoping she was making a good choice. When the margins came back clean, but very narrow, she wondered anew about her prognosis and asked her surgeon if she should go back in and widen the margins just a bit. "Can't we do another lumpectomy?" she proposed.

"That's not in the protocol," the surgeon told her. "It gets harder and harder to get to the same area if we do repeated lumpectomies. That risks having the breast not look good, which is the whole point of a lumpectomy."

"What about the risk?" asked Susan.

"The statistics show that clean margins are clean margins, even if they're only clean by less than a millimeter."

"So, I either have a mastectomy or I make my peace with narrow margins?"

"Yes," nodded the surgeon.

Susan sighed and started radiation treatment.

More Art Than Science

The next decision involved tamoxifen. A five-year hormonal inter-vention, tamoxifen decreases a woman's risk of recurrence or metas-tasis, but wreaks havoc on her hormones and can cause menopauselike symptoms. Most troubling to Susan, it isn't safe to get pregnant while taking tamoxifen because of potential risk to the fetus.

Susan felt she had had enough trouble finding a husband when she was in her thirties and healthy; now she was forty and a cancer patient, a diagnosis that could make her unattractive to a potential mate. And tamoxifen would give her menopausal-like sweats and mood swings. And if she took tamoxifen until she was forty-five, when her fertility would drop yet again and chances of birth defects would rise, the cancer might have robbed her of children as well. She wasn't sure she liked her choices: increased risk of recurrence or expe-riencing the effects of menopause and a life without children. Going into "pseudo-menopause" at age forty, Susan felt, would be like los-ing ten years of her life.

Susan wasn't sure if fertility was possible at her age, or if it was prudent after breast cancer. Reading one scientific article after another, she found that women who have had breast cancer and then gotten pregnant have no greater chance of recurrence or metastasis than women who haven't gotten pregnant. Changes in the breast caused by a full-term pregnancy can protect somewhat against breast cancer, and women who have never had children have a slightly higher risk of getting breast cancer than women who have. Researchers also found that breast cancer survivors who did have a recurrence within two to three years after having a baby had a worse prognosis than women who weren't recently pregnant. But women who survived for seven or eight years after diagnosis benefited from the protective effect of pregnancy; changes in the breast that support lactation also make it less likely to have a recurrence of cancer.

As she was grappling with this decision, Susan reluctantly went to a breast cancer survivors' conference to learn more about the disease, tamoxifen, and fertility. But when she set foot into the room full of young survivors, her outlook changed. The women were all surviving and vibrant and, most important of all, *young*. Susan was actually one of the oldest survivors in the room. She was exhilarated. That room, those women and their vitality, gave Susan back the decade of her life she felt she had lost.

With this renewed sense of possibilities came fresh concerns about tamoxifen. Susan hit the books and the Internet and found that tamoxifen was originally developed as a fertility agent. In addition, while use of tamoxifen lowered the chances of breast cancer a great deal, it also slightly boosted the possibility of uterine cancer. The notion is that the decreased risk of breast cancer outweighs the increased chances of uterine cancer.

"This is where medicine became more art than science," Susan told a friend. "It isn't binary, on-off, black-white." She decided to collect a few opinions.

Her radiation oncologist said that she should have at least some tamoxifen. She could take it for two years, then go off the drug and have a child. But he had no idea what effect tamoxifen would have on her reproductive system, nor how long it would take for her body to revert to pre-tamoxifen status.

Another oncologist said she would very much like to see Susan on tamoxifen, but suggested she delay it for a year or two, to "resolve the child issue."

A third suggested that tamoxifen wasn't as critical for Susan as for other young women. Yes, tamoxifen reduces the risk of recurrence or metastasis, but given Susan's diagnosis, the chances of recurrence were pretty small to start with, and cutting a pretty small percentage in half was simply making something that was very small into something even smaller.

A conservative breast cancer researcher wasn't fazed at all by the idea of a DCIS survivor getting pregnant. Would a pregnancy mean that a recurrence would be more likely to be invasive than in situ, or DCIS?

"We don't know. We don't know that it would, we don't know that it wouldn't," she said. "We just don't know."

Breast cancer specialists were fairly consistent. They supported women getting pregnant after breast cancer, but thought that fertility medications were a bad idea, because taking them required boosting a woman's estrogen level for a few months.

Fertility specialists pointed out that pregnancy itself boosted a woman's estrogen level even higher than fertility drugs and for a longer period of time; if pregnancy was safe, then what was the matter with fertility meds? Another one of those tricky questions, Susan decided.

Ultimately, Susan realized that there probably wasn't any more science to unearth. But the more people she talked to, the more different approaches and views she heard. She talked to people who were much more conservative in their approaches and people who were much more relaxed about it. Oncologists and fertility specialists view the situation through different lenses and come to different conclusions. Oncologists were saying okay to pregnancy but not to fertility meds; fertility specialists were saying that if pregnancy is all right, then why not also fertility meds?

How Could She Give Up?

The most conservative oncologist, who had a reputation for being patient-centered, asked a disturbing question: "How likely is it that you would have children anyway?" Susan never determined whether he was referring to her age, the fact that she was single, or something else. He went on to discuss the need to give up a dream that might not be realistic. Not everyone could ski the Alps or fly to the moon, he said. If a dream was unlikely to happen, if she realized that it was unlikely, then perhaps it would be easier to give it up. And if she was going to give up on the dream of having children, then why couldn't she just take tamoxifen for the recommended five years? It would offer her the maximum amount of protection available.

Susan was stunned. How could someone equate having a child, that most basic of human instincts and needs, with flying to the moon? How could he suggest that it was as easy to "give up" on having a child as to give up on becoming an astronaut?

After that appointment, Susan headed straight home. She tried to remind herself that this doctor had worked in oncology for years and had seen too many women die. As a result of spending his career trying to save women's lives, he had become particularly conservative. She told herself that it was for this very perspective that she went to see him, to explore the full range of opinion on fertility and breast cancer, but it didn't help. When she got home, Susan slammed her front door, threw her keys on the floor, and crashed onto her sofa where she cried, and wailed, and raged. She felt more anger than she'd ever felt before. Fuming, she grabbed an old pillow and a pair of scissors and proceeded to stab the pillow over and over. She destroyed that pillow the way the oncologist had unintentionally destroyed her dreams of family.

But family was what Susan wanted most in her post-cancer life. No matter how hard she tried to redirect her thoughts, they always came back to marriage, family, and children. Before her diagnosis, she'd been upset about not having them. Then breast cancer came along and took her mind off it. It was like going on vacation; you come back and all your old problems are still there. It was as though she went away to breast cancer and then came back to her old life. What did she want in her post-cancer life, her "second chance?" The same two things she had wanted before diagnosis: marriage and children. Marriage could happen at any time, she reminded herself; children were time-limited.

She spoke with other single people who started families on their own and realized that if she were married she would take the plunge. She would be doing everything in her power to get pregnant.

When she read other survivors' stories of breast cancer, many of them expressed gratitude for their families. "They say they never would have made it if it weren't for their husbands, for their children," she told a friend. "I wish I had that."

Among her piles and piles of notes, Susan came across a phone number for a reproductive endocrinologist—a fertility expert. She slipped the number into her purse to call the next day.

Single Parenting

"This is my situation," Susan began. "I'm facing a decision about tamoxifen and I'm forty years old and I'm trying to understand where I am in my fertility." Susan explained her situation in more detail. The doctor understood it, respected her feelings, and was sympathetic. For the first time, Susan felt that a medical professional really heard what she was saying.

Yes, he explained, certain blood tests could indicate whether she might still be able to get pregnant. It wasn't foolproof, he said. "The blood work can look lousy and people can still get pregnant. The blood work can look good and people still can't get pregnant. Especially older women. But, yes, there is a way to see where you are hormonally."

Susan felt as though she had empowered herself. She didn't know what effect the information would have. If the odds were low that she would get pregnant, would she give it up and start the tamoxifen? She just didn't know.

When Susan went back to the office for the results, the reproductive endocrinologist told her, "You're not in bad shape for a woman of your age. The blood work is within the normal ranges, but there's no guarantee. Even with good blood work it's still harder to get pregnant in your forties than earlier."

"So I could have a child?" Susan gasped. Finally, irrefutable evidence that having a baby was not completely out of the question.

"If you wanted to conceive a child, I'd be willing to work with you," he continued. Susan gasped and grabbed at the armrest of her chair, certain that her physical equilibrium was as startled as her emotional state. Could she do it as a single woman? Could she get over the stigma of something so nontraditional? Could she work out the logistics? She knew plenty of married women who had a hard time juggling career and child-rearing. And what about her finances? She worked in the computer industry, which was going through tremendous upheavals in the early twenty-first century, with layoffs every other quarter. Could she count on keeping her job? What about her social life? She tried to imagine bringing a baby to a fancy restaurant. Would having a child completely ruin her chances of ever getting married?

"What about the risks to my body?" Susan asked.

"There are no guarantees. It depends on how you feel about taking risks," said the doctor. "How do you feel about riding in small planes? About riding motorcycles?" he asked. "How do you feel about taking risks that are risks, but seem reasonable risks?"

That perspective revolutionized Susan's thinking. It wasn't a question of risk or no risk. It was an issue of how much risk she felt comfortable with. She realized that she had no guarantees either way. She could have a recurrence if she got pregnant, she could have a recurrence if she didn't. The cancer could recur whether she fulfilled her dream or not. And it wasn't just cancer. She could get hit by a car any day of the week. There are no guarantees in this life. So, if there are no guarantees, and it doesn't seem like an overly high risk, why not do what her heart really wanted? There was no question that having a child was what her heart really wanted.

Susan went to a meeting of Single Mothers by Choice, an organization of single women who had become parents through either pregnancy or adoption. All the women she met there were caring, intelligent professionals, mostly in their thirties and forties. They simply weren't married, and didn't want to or thought they couldn't continue to wait and decided to start their own families. Susan found it inspiring. It made single parenting by choice seem less radical, less weird, and more normal. It made single parenting seem like something she could do.

Susan decided that, yes, she wanted to bear a child. Her parents worried about what it might mean for her survival, but were thrilled at the thought of another grandchild. And the people in her workplace had been very supportive. Everyone who knew how much Susan wanted a family was excited for her.

Nine Beautiful Pounds

In April 2003, Susan gave birth to nine-pound Diana. Susan took one look at her daughter and started to cry. "I never knew anyone could be so beautiful," she whispered to Diana. "I never knew I could love anyone this much."

Susan had a rough time getting started with nursing. The breast that had been treated didn't produce much milk and the untreated breast had a very flat nipple that bled whenever Diana sucked. But Susan was determined to make breast-feeding work. With a little practice, Diana became a voracious breast-feeder and their marathon nursing sessions became a special bonding time for mother and daughter. But it disturbs Susan to think that whenever Diana goes for checkups, she is going to have to tell her doctor that her mother had breast cancer. It increases her risk for the disease and is a part of her own medical record.

Susan's new life has enhanced her awareness that there's no such thing as "no risk." "Until I was diagnosed with breast cancer, I never thought of myself as being seriously at risk for health issues. I never had to make decisions like whether I should take a drug that will increase my risk of one cancer in order to decrease my risk of another cancer. When life starts to look like that, you realize that you're living in a world of risks. At the same time, no one told me that it was medically unsound to get pregnant. If anyone had said it was a risk they would not approve of, I would have not gotten pregnant and dealt with the situation. I just hope and pray that I chose wisely. I hope and I pray that I made a prudent decision and that neither Diana nor I will suffer for it."

In her more nervous moments, Susan yearns for a simple, normal life. But in a strange way, she owes her smiling, cooing complication to another, less adorable one. If it hadn't been for breast cancer, Susan thinks, she might never have been catapulted into action. If she hadn't realized how strongly she wanted a family, how adamantly she believed it was an important goal—not a frivolous and unrealistic dream—she might never have taken steps to make it happen. And she wouldn't be watching and applauding Diana's efforts to blow raspberries.

"I am not grateful that I had breast cancer," she explains, "but I do think that I used the experience to change my life. I reacted to it in good ways as well as in difficult ones. Sometimes it seems weird to say that it feels like a blessing. Because why do I deserve a blessing more than anyone else?" she asks. "But Diana is here and she's wonderful. Now there are days when I leave work and my heart sings. I'm overjoyed because I'm going to get my daughter at day care. All of a sudden, I have something to come home to. She's wonderful and she fills my life and my heart in a way nothing else has."

Susan was recently laid off in another computer-industry blip. She and Diana have taken the opportunity to spend more time together. She is in good health now.

☐ ☐ ☐

Many young women find they want to have children after fighting breast cancer. Part of the reason is to pick up the pieces of their lives. But it can also be life-affirming. As Susan explains, "It was what I wanted to do with my second chance." And it was particularly important to have her own child, if it was medically possible and safe for both her and the child.

Roberta agreed. She knew she'd always wanted to have children. When she met Lee, whom she dated during treatment and then married, she realized she "wanted him to be reproduced." She researched the question and realized that the data showed no additional risk as a result of pregnancy after breast cancer. She closed her eyes one day on a walk and decided, "Let's go for it." Though she worried about whether she would be around for the child's formative years, it wasn't a huge concern. Roberta had grown up without a father and still felt very lucky. She knew that even if she didn't live, her children—she now has two daughters—would be "the luckiest kids in the world."

WHAT IF I WANT TO ADOPT?

꿏ᰫ Jacquie,* 29: A Different Life, a Parallel Life

NORMALLY, FLYING DIDN'T BOTHER JACQUIE, but this time she was nauseated the entire trip. She looked around the half-filled 747 and noticed that no one else was visibly ill. Even the little children on the flight seemed antsy, but not uncomfortable. As she perused the aisles, she also saw that she was the only African American on the plane.

A series of unrelated questions whirred through her brain. She worried about her husband, Mitch. His recent brain surgery had turned up a benign tumor, but he had seemed uncharacteristically lethargic since. A lawyer for the state of North Carolina, Mitch was usually full of energy. Jacquie wondered how she was going to organize the latest get-out-the-vote campaign she had volunteered to spearhead for the local Democratic party. She could hear the voice of the latest woman to join the battered women's shelter she ran; despite her social work training and years of counseling experience, she often got caught up in graphic descriptions of abuse. And she worried about getting home in time for her hair appointment; she was going to end up with an Afro if she wasn't careful.

She wondered about her future. Should she apply to that MBA program, the one with the concentration in organizational development? That would shock her friends, who were sure she was going for a political career, but her work at her nonprofit service organization had really piqued her interest in administration. And what about having a child? She and Mitch, both twenty-nine, had just begun talking about whether there were kids in their future.

Jacquie felt her stomach lurch and she looked around the plane again; perhaps there was something going on with *her*. She pulled a mirror from her purse and straightened her collar. The rose dress, from the local seven-dollar store, complemented her walnut-colored skin nicely. If she was going to feel miserable, then at least she was going to look good.

*Not her real name

When she arrived home, she scheduled a trip to her gynecologist, who later confirmed her suspicions: She *was* pregnant.

At first, Jacquie was ambivalent. She wasn't sure whether she wanted a child, whether this was a good time in her career to make such a radical change. And what about graduate school? Would she have to give up her ambitions, as so many other women did when they became mothers?

One evening, Jacquie and Mitch went for an after-dinner walk in their suburban neighborhood just outside of Raleigh. The late-summer heat had cooled a bit and a pleasant breeze was blowing. Children played in a paved driveway nearby, some kids rode by on bikes, and several young couples were out pushing infants in strollers. As they strolled the sidewalk, they wondered whether the baby would be a girl or a boy. "I've been thinking about the name Amanda," Mitch proposed. Jacquie surprised herself by nodding. They wondered whether the child would like soccer or basketball, what school subjects he or she would excel in. They considered decorating schemes to turn the guest bedroom into a nursery. Slowly, Jacquie warmed to the idea of having a child; she began to look forward to the third member of their little family.

A few months later, as the leaves started to fall, the board of directors of the child-abuse prevention organization that Jacquie ran decided to merge with a domestic violence program. The two boards picked a name for the new organization and decided to start by laying off everyone in both organizations. Then they would hire an executive director and let the new director select the rest of the staff, with the understanding that former staffers would be employed if a position matched their skills and experience. Jacquie decided to interview for the new position.

The interviews were held at a local law office, where one of the board members worked. Jacquie had never been in the building before and when she arrived, just after grabbing a quick lunch, she made a pit stop in the ladies' room for a bout of morning sickness that still hadn't learned to tell time. As she rinsed her mouth and crunched a few saltines to settle her stomach, Jacquie decided to tell the interviewers that she was pregnant. She knew she didn't legally have to. She and Mitch had decided not to spread the word until after her first trimester, so friends and family didn't even know yet. But it seemed the only honorable move.

The interview went well, and as it drew to a close, Jacquie disclosed her condition.

"By the way, I'm pregnant. I'm due in June and would plan to take the summer off." She paused, surveying the still-friendly faces. "I thought you ought to figure that information into your decision."

A few days later, Jacquie was offered the Executive Director position. It was the middle of October and the merger was effective January 1.

Setting an Appointment

In December, at the end of Jacquie's first trimester, the nausea dissipated. She became more comfortable with the changes that were happening to her body and found herself touching her breasts frequently.

One day, she felt a lump. First, she panicked; wasn't that a sign of cancer? But then she relaxed and decided that she was too young for such a diagnosis. It must be a benign cyst, a clogged gland, or a gland developing. Some innocuous pregnancy-related phenomenon that would be sorted out if only she would remember to ask her doctor. It took a few weeks before Jacquie posed the question.

"I think you ought to get this checked out," her doctor said, once he located the lump.

"Okay, sure." Jacquie took off her glasses to pull her shirt over her head.

"I think you ought to get this checked out right away," he repeated.

Jacquie tucked her blue blouse into her flowered skirt and slung her pocketbook over her shoulder. "Okay, sure."

The obstetrician cleared his throat. "Let's make an appointment for you, before you leave, to have someone take a look at this."

Jacquie sat back down and stared at the doctor. "You've got my attention now. Why do I need to see someone immediately?"

"It's a little unusual," the obstetrician replied. "You should have it checked out."

The doctor asked his nurse to set an appointment with a breast surgeon. Then he turned to Jacquie apologetically. "From your reaction, I didn't have any confidence that you would call by yourself—or even if you did, I figured you probably wouldn't call soon enough." He told Jacquie that the surgeon would probably do a needle biopsy.

During that week, Jacquie began spotting. Her obstetrician confirmed her worst fear. The sonogram showed that the fetus had died. Jacquie was devastated. She hadn't set out to have a child—it had come to her. "It was a gift," she told Mitch. "And gifts shouldn't be taken away." Unless it was because she hadn't wanted the child enough at first. Surely she hadn't caused the miscarriage. Whatever the reason, Jacquie was inconsolable.

The needle biopsy performed a few days later proved inconclusive. She would need an incisional biopsy. The surgeon would remove some of the lump and test it for cancer; they would then know if she needed further surgery.

"Cancer is a possibility," said the surgeon. "But you're twenty-nine years old and you don't fit the profile of someone who would have breast cancer. You don't have any risk factors that we know of." Jacquie was adopted, so she didn't know all the details of her family history. She wasn't really worried about breast cancer; that was a disease that hit older women. She was thinking about her lost child.

When she woke up from the anesthesia, she was greeted by her breast surgeon. "You have cancer," he said.

People get cancer and die, Jacquie thought. They die quickly or they die slowly. But someone gets cancer and moves into the final stage of her life.

She felt wronged by the diagnosis. She'd been a good person, she'd spent her life trying to help children and their families. Then, within a span of just a few months, her husband had survived a brain tumor, she'd gotten pregnant and then miscarried, and now she had breast cancer. Jacquie never questioned whether the cancer had played a role in her miscarriage. She didn't ask, and no one ever mentioned it. Perhaps on some level, she didn't want to know the answer.

Getting Her Body Working Again

Jacquie didn't want to learn about different forms of surgery, she didn't want to hear about chemotherapy or radiology. She wasn't even curious about nutrition and vitamins. She just wanted to get the cancer *out* of her body. Immediately.

But the biopsy didn't do the trick; there was more cancer left in her body. Jacquie was admitted to the hospital right after her incisional-biopsy surgery. The very next day, she had a modified radical Halsted mastectomy to remove the rest of the cancer. Jacquie wouldn't know until later, but her cancer was advanced. She had stage III cancer, which had moved into her lymph nodes and had affected all but one. The surgeon had removed the tumor and breast tissue, scraped the muscle tissue, and taken out all of her lymph nodes. Faced with a choice, Jacquie knew she wasn't ready to think about any more surgery, so she opted for using a prosthesis rather than reconstructive surgery on her breast.

Once Jacquie could take care of her basic needs, she was discharged from the hospital, a week before Christmas. Her medical condition and psychological state put a damper on what was usually a very festive time for the couple. Neither Mitch nor Jacquie had the energy to get a large tree, as they usually did, or to hang the traditional lights or wreaths that typically adorned the house. Mitch retrieved an artificial tabletop tree from the back of the garage.

On Christmas Day, Mitch put on a new sweater that Jacquie had gotten for him, but Jacquie never even changed out of her pajamas. "They fit comfortably over my bandages," she explained. They avoided the large family celebrations they usually attended and had a quiet Christmas breakfast, just the two of them.

"Don't Tell Me"

Jacquie was grateful that she was out of commission during the winter holidays so her absence was not conspicuous. When she returned to the office in January, she tried to put her staff at ease. "What do you think of my new hairstyle?" she joked, pointing to her short bob. She had cut her hair in anticipation of losing it during chemotherapy. Then she changed the subject and never went back to it. No one on her staff asked any questions; it was as though someone had warned them to avoid the subject.

After the holidays, Jacquie started an aggressive regimen of chemotherapy. She took two days off each time she had chemotherapy, one day for the treatment itself and a second to recuperate. She realized that her oncologist would tell her what she wanted to know, but only if she asked. She didn't want her oncologist to "slip" and give her more information than she had specifically requested. Most days, she just wanted to know where she had to be and when.

But she never wanted to know her prognosis.

Eventually Jacquie found that she did want to know a little more about her disease. She walked into her oncologist's office with a list of questions.

"It took me years to learn what I know about breast cancer," the doctor said. "Do you want to know what I know?" She nodded. He brought out a massive textbook and handed it over. She dutifully carried it home, left it in the backseat of her car, and brought it back at her next appointment. She hadn't so much as cracked the binding. She found a slimmer and less intimidating volume from the American Cancer Society. She read on the days when she felt strong and forgot the information on those days when she didn't want to know it.

During chemo, Jacquie created elaborate games to gauge her progress. If the doctor smiled at her, it meant that he was hopeful that she was going to be all right. If he didn't interact with her, then it meant that he saw her as a patient. If she was a patient to him, she was going to die. If she could be a real person to him, if he made an investment in her as a person, he thought she was going to live. This was a game, a game that kept her going, kept her strong, kept her sealed off from the emotions of the experience.

꙰

Central North Carolina gets New England–style snow only every five or six years. One of those years was 1981. That February was also the month Jacquie lost her hair. Within forty-eight hours, her neighborhood was covered with nearly a foot of snow and Jacquie had lost so much hair she wasn't sure she could *ever* leave home. She hadn't realized how much her long, wavy hair had been a part of her identity.

By the time Mitch dug the car out, Jacquie had put a scarf on her head and decided to go shopping for a wig. After a few false starts, she found an "ethnic" shop downtown that had a fairly good selection of wigs. She decided to have fun with her hairpieces. She chose a Donna Summer disco wig and a sophisticated Stefanie Powers wig for her more corporate moods. But she wanted one more.

"Ever since I was a child, I've always been Pocahontas in my dreams," Jacquie told Mitch. So she bought a Pocahontas wig with two thick black braids. She had managed to turn her depressing baldness into an opportunity to live out an innocent, silly dream.

The prosthesis, too, took some adjustment. But with minor changes to her wardrobe, Jacquie felt better about her appearance. It was a relief to look at herself in the mirror and see that she looked okay. After all, if she looked okay, she could convince herself that she *was* okay. She'd been raised to believe that looking good wasn't just half the battle, it was at least 75 percent.

But every night, Jacquie took off her costume. She draped her wig on its Styrofoam stand and saw her bald head. Then she took off her prosthesis and saw the scar racing across her chest.

Trying THC

For Jacquie, handling chemotherapy meant being able to work and take care of the house. In that sense, she tolerated treatment well. She received chemo every three weeks for nearly eleven months. Since no family or friends, not even Mitch, accompanied Jacquie to chemo, a nurse or medical assistant often sat with her while she received the treatment. She felt the medical staff took a special interest in her because she was an anomaly, being so young.

Nausea was a constant nuisance. One day, Jacquie asked her oncologist for a prescription for tetrahydrocannabinol (THC), the active ingredient in marijuana, which she thought was medically indicated. She didn't want to get high, she wanted to avoid the nausea.

"It's not going to feel like you think it will," the doctor said. "It's not the same as smoking it." But Jacquie was certain he was holding out on her. She continued to make the request and eventually got a prescription.

THC is a controlled substance, so Jacquie had to go to a medical center pharmacy to get the prescription filled. She parked in the huge asphalt lot, entered the massive doors, and walked down the corridors to the pharmacy, resentful that she couldn't pick it up in her local drugstore. She pushed open the swinging door to the dispensary.

A prenatal class had just let out and participants were picking up their multivitamins. The pharmacy was filled with pregnant women, ranging from just-beginning-to-show to about-to-go-into-labor. Jacquie's eyes zeroed in on the adolescents, who seemed to take over the room. They have no business being pregnant, Jacquie thought as she wove her way through the protruding bellies to the counter. They're too young to be pregnant. They probably don't even want to have a baby. And they can probably get pregnant again if they want to. I should be pregnant right now, she thought. But I'm not. And after all this chemotherapy, who knows if I'll ever be able to get pregnant again. By the time Jacquie paid for her prescription and had the vial in hand, she was consumed with anger.

Making No Plans

Jacquie was depressed most of the time that she was on chemotherapy. She was exhausted from the chemo, from her demanding job, and from just trying to hold herself together. Jacquie's notion of a "good day" changed; a good day during this period would have seemed substandard just a few months earlier. Jacquie felt as though her life had been turned upside down. She had been in control, a successful young woman. Then everything changed, through no fault of her own. Her body had betrayed her. Cancer was something she could never prevent nor control, and if it happened once, it could happen again and she wouldn't even know until it was too late.

During this time, Jacquie didn't talk to her oncologist; it took all of her emotional energy just to show up for her appointments. She didn't remember her questions when she walked into the office or his answers when she walked out. In what felt like a final humiliation, she began writing down her questions and his responses. This, she thought, was what breast cancer did to a woman in control. It left her unable to remember even the most important information.

Jacquie's life became very narrow. She would wake up, shower and dress mechanically, and focus on composing and crossing off items on her list of tasks for the day. Before the cancer diagnosis, Jacquie had always acted with an eye toward her long-term goals. But now she stopped making plans—plans for next year or the following month, even lunch dates for the following week.

She adopted a dress-for-success model. If she acknowledged how sick she was, she would actually become that sick. If she acted better than she felt, if she told people she felt better than she really did, she would start to feel the way she acted. Jacquie tried to do it all alone. She met periodically with a Reach to Recovery volunteer, whom Jacquie thought of as elderly. All they had in common, Jacquie felt, was breast cancer, and that just wasn't enough. She also went to a monthly support group at the local women's center, but there were no young women in it. She didn't talk to her friends or family. One evening, during chemotherapy, Jacquie and her best friend, Karen, met to chat and ended up in an all-night Hardee's, sipping sodas and munching on french fries. They started out griping about Karen's latest ill-fated relationship. Then they turned to Jacquie's troubles. "I feel maimed, I feel disfigured," she said. "All my plans—school, children, career, every-thing—are out the window. And there's nothing I can do about it, no way I could have predicted it. It's just so unfair. My body betrayed me and I can't even find all the pieces, much less pick them up."

That evening, Jacquie felt cleansed and refreshed. It was the first and only time she talked about her frustration. Despite her counseling background, she was surprised how good it felt. Even so, she never permitted herself that luxury again.

๛

As soon as Jacquie's body recuperated from chemotherapy, about a year after the mastectomy, she had her left breast reconstructed using a saline implant. The plastic surgeon performed it in a same-day surgery clinic. He suggested that Jacquie stay overnight, but she wanted to go home. Patients stay in a hospital, she thought, and she didn't want to be a patient. Jacquie decided that she didn't want to have her nipple reconstructed. Her goal was simple: Get rid of the prosthesis. It slipped around too much; it was too uncomfortable. But she didn't need the nipple; its absence would be a daily reminder of the challenges she had overcome and the challenges she would continue to face.

Starting to Have Fun

It took about seven or eight months after chemo until Jacquie's hair was mostly grown back. When she could run her fingers through her even-curlier tresses, she began to put her life back together, although she still couldn't plan ahead. She and Mitch began going to clubs. They would decide, sometimes as late as ten o'clock at night, to go dancing. They'd just hop into the car and head out. It was a social life that they'd never had before. Mitch seemed mildly surprised but amenable; they never actually discussed the change.

Slowly, Jacquie started having fun. At first, she could go for a few hours without thinking about breast cancer, then she went for a day or two. Eventually, she could go for a week without thinking about it. But then it would be time for her three-month checkup and she would have to confront the disease again.

Jacquie and Mitch also began trying to conceive again, but it soon became clear that the chemotherapy had so sapped Jacquie's reproductive system that she was not going to be able to get pregnant again. They began to think about adopting a baby girl.

Adoption didn't worry Jacquie. She herself had been adopted, so she'd always considered it a viable possibility. But she was concerned about becoming a parent. She wasn't sure she'd be around to see a child through life's important milestones: first grade, high school graduation, marriage. She wasn't even convinced she'd be able to see her child's first step or hear her first words. Jacquie's father had died when she was eighteen, so she felt that her daughter would be moving into adulthood at that age and could take care of herself if necessary. But it was very important to Jacquie that she be around for her daughter for those first eighteen years.

Finally, Jacquie convinced herself that she could start the adoption process and get all the way to the point of meeting the child. But if at any point it became too painful, she could just stop it. She didn't mention her insecurities to Mitch, but she struck a deal with herself: If they ever brought a baby into the house, she would be committed to it. But up to that point, she would allow herself to change her mind.

Jacquie called the Children's Home Society, which put her and Mitch on a list for the next information session. But then the society found out that they were African American and called them in for a meeting the following week. They were having a difficult time finding homes for black children and were pleased to find a young, professional couple eager to adopt.

Jacquie and Mitch began the process: They read the required parenting materials, wrote their biographical sketches, gave names of friends and family to be interviewed as character references, and spoke with the caseworker multiple times. Jacquie was pleasant enough during these conversations, but she was resentful. She couldn't stop thinking about the pregnant adolescents in the medical center pharmacy; they didn't have to apply to anyone, didn't have to study, didn't have to prove themselves. Why should *she* have to? Silently, Jacquie spent her time critiquing the caseworker's interviewing technique. But she was careful, she thought, to hide her cynicism.

She mentioned that she'd survived breast cancer in an offhand manner that, she hoped, would not jeopardize the adoption. She wanted to be honest, but tried to run her life as though she'd never had the disease. She didn't want breast cancer to take any more from her than it already had.

Jacquie and Mitch were approved for adoption.

The caseworker had interviewed various friends and family members, including Karen. Later, Karen told Jacquie that she'd been asked, "So, what's with Jacquie? Why is she so aloof? Does she really want to adopt a child?"

Thirty-six Days Old

The society warned Jacquie and Mitch that it might take up to three years to find a child for them. They added that it might be quicker if the couple was willing to take a biracial child. African American families want African American children, white families want white children, Indian families want Indian children; biracial kids have no natural constituency. Jacquie is biracial herself, so she had no problem with that. They agreed to adopt an African American or biracial child, signed the pertinent papers, and went home.

Jacquie and Mitch were approved for adoption in March. By Easter, they started preparing the nursery, and propped a Cabbage Patch doll in the crib.

Their caseworker called Jacquie at work on the Tuesday after Easter. "You have a baby girl," she said. "She's a month old. You can meet her tomorrow, if you like."

That night, Jacquie raced to meet Mitch at the children's section in Sears. They positioned themselves in the middle of the infant section, found a saleswoman, and started pointing. They picked out three onesies, three receiving blankets, several baby-sized towels and wash-cloths, a hat, several pairs of socks and stockings, and a dressy outfit for that exciting first trip home. Then they picked out a car seat, unsure how to install it but certain that it was necessary.

By the time Jacquie and Mitch got home, there were packages from friends and relatives waiting on the front porch. They never did figure out how everyone knew. As they walked into their living room, Jacquie was stricken with panic. She was about to make a lifelong commit-ment to a child. How could she be sure this was the right child? Would a smile be a good sign? she wondered. Can a thirty-five-day-old infant even smile at all, or would a set of upturned lips just be a sign of gas? Jacquie decided that she wouldn't know for sure if this was the right child. But, she figured, she'd feel in her gut if it was the wrong one.

The next day, Jacquie and Mitch walked into their caseworker's office and saw a cinnamon-colored, nearly bald infant, dressed in an ornate christening gown, asleep in a pink bassinet on the case-worker's desk. Jacquie drew her breath in and stared as Mitch went over to touch a lacy bootie. As Jacquie slowly exhaled, she tentatively caressed the right side of the baby's face.

"This is Jas, short for Jasmine," said the caseworker in a quiet voice.

"She's beautiful," Jacquie said, experiencing an assortment of emo-tions: joy, terror, calm, and a sense of overwhelming responsibility. But she had no feeling that she couldn't do it, no sense that Jas wasn't the "right one." Jas woke with a gurgle and Jacquie plucked her out of the bassinet. Mitch handed Jacquie the pink flowered dress and white ruffled tights that had seemed perfectly practical in the check-out line at Sears.

Jas squirmed and wriggled as any baby might, and Jacquie could barely keep up; she had never even babysat as a teenager and hadn't really known what to expect. Eventually, she got the child dressed by pinning down one wiggly little leg at a time. The caseworker helped the couple install the car seat into the middle of the backseat, and assisted in positioning Jas. They drove off, conscious of every bump in the road.

Adopting a child, for Jacquie, meant being able to think about the future with some confidence. That day in Greensboro, Jacquie made an eighteen-year commitment to Jas.

A Parallel Life

Every year, Jacquie picks up another thread she dropped when she heard the diagnosis "breast cancer." She began working in academia and earned her doctorate. But she made a major detour from the life she had thought she would lead. While she gets closer and closer her new goals, it is with some regrets. Regrets that her career hasn't gone as she had originally planned. Regrets that motherhood came later and differently than she had hoped. Regrets that her educational plans were delayed and then changed.

And she feels disfigured. She's always aware, even sixteen years after diagnosis, that when she goes clothes shopping, she must buy shirts that hide the fact that one breast is not real. She never wears tight-fitting T-shirts; she hates bathing suits. She doesn't like any-one—even Mitch—to see her body. She doesn't wear slinky lingerie and prefers to make love with the lights out.

She loves her husband, her daughter, her career, and her home. But her days are peppered with moments of wistfulness and bitterness. Jacquie sees herself, now, as back on course, but with different per-spectives, different choices, different options. A parallel path. Not the one she expected from life, but another one, moving forward.

Jacquie now holds a doctorate in adult education and works as a college administrator. She lives in central North Carolina with her husband and their teenage daughter, Jasmine. Jacquie is closing in on her eighteen-year commitment to her daughter.

◻ ◻ ◻

Some young women decide to adopt a child after breast cancer because the treatment, as with Jacquie, has left them no alternative.

Indeed, Becky required her fiancé to agree to the possibility of adoption as a condition of marriage. Other young women, though, choose adoption for health reasons. Helen, for instance, has chosen to start the adoption process because she worries about the effect of pregnancy on an estrogen-receptor-positive cancer and is afraid childbirth will contribute to a recurrence or metastasis. Dana and Lanita also decided to adopt, although for a different health reason. Both worried about the health of their children.

WHAT IF I HAVE CHILDREN?

✺⟡ Barbara, 26: Telling the Girls

BARBARA LAY IN BED THE NIGHT SHE WAS DIAGNOSED with breast cancer, trying to figure out how to tell her children. They were so different. Brooke, eight years old, was focused on school and her friends. At four, Lacey was much less independent, much more focused on home. Who should tell them, me or Leo? What should I say? How will they react? Barbara wondered.

She felt her own mortality. Will I live to see them graduate high school? Will I even see their next birthdays? If I don't make it, who is going to raise them? Who will make sure Lacey has milk money? Who will check Brooke's homework? Are they going to have a stepmother? Would someone replace me? I don't want anyone else taking care of my children. I don't want anyone trying to take my place. She started to cry, thinking, I'm never going to see my daughters graduate. I'm never going to watch them walk down the aisle.

Every morning, Barbara got up with the girls while her husband, Leo, slept. She got them fed and dressed and bundled Brooke off to the bus stop just a few blocks from their home in suburban Maine. Then the van came to pick up Lacey and take her to preschool. Barbara enjoyed this morning time with the girls because once they came home from school, she had to head out to the local factory, where she worked second shift on the assembly line, making electronic components. By that time, Leo was up, rested from his third shift at a different factory.

The arrangement was ideal, Barbara thought, because both parents got to spend lots of quality time with the kids. The girls were rarely, if ever, with a babysitter.

Days flowed smoothly. Barbara and Leo figured the hard times were over. They'd survived teen parenthood and dropping out of high school. They had married when Brooke was eighteen months old. Three and a half years later, Lacey was born, and the family was almost complete. They had planned on one more child, and both of them, especially Leo, hoped it would be a boy, to carry on the family name.

One weekend in February, Barbara was shaving under her arms and felt something unusual. She put down the razor and proceeded to do a breast self-examination, making careful circles with her fingertips. She felt a pealike lump in her left breast, so small it was barely noticeable. When she mentioned it casually to Leo, he urged her to call a doctor immediately.

The family doctor asked Barbara to come in the next day for a checkup. "I think we should do a mammogram," he said.

"But I'm only twenty-six," Barbara said. "Aren't I too young for anything serious? Don't you think it's just a cyst?"

"We should do a mammogram to rule out anything bad," said the doctor. "We can do it right now, if you're ready." Barbara looked over at Leo, who nodded. Barbara took a deep breath and smiled at the doctor.

The Birthday Party

When Barbara called for the results of the test two days later, the nurse wouldn't say anything, just told her that the doctor would return the call. Barbara didn't understand why the nurse couldn't tell her the results. When the doctor finally called, a few hours later, he told her that she was awfully young. And that he had made an appointment for her the following week to see a breast surgeon he recommended. Barbara felt even more confused and a little worried.

Leo went with Barbara to the surgeon. Barbara kept saying, as though it was a mantra, "I'm too young to have breast cancer. This is benign. I'm too young."

When they walked into the examination room, the surgeon held up Barbara's mammogram to the light and pointed out the calcifications. "You probably have breast cancer," he told her bluntly.

Barbara felt her heart plummet to the floor. I'm going to die, she thought.

"We need to do a biopsy to be sure," the surgeon continued.

Then Barbara's fear turned to anger. "What if I just walk out this door right now?" she demanded. "My little girl's birthday is next weekend. What if I just leave now?"

"If you walk out this door," the surgeon said in a quiet voice, "you will not be around for your daughter's next birthday."

Barbara was silent.

"There are two ways to test the lump," the surgeon continued, looking straight at Leo. "We could aspirate it, but the results wouldn't be definitive. We could also do a biopsy, where we extract some of the tissue and test it; that way, we would know for sure what is going on. If it were my wife," he said, still staring at Leo and avoiding Barbara's eyes, "I would go with the biopsy."

Barbara waved at the surgeon to get his attention. "It's *my* body we're talking about. *I* get to make the decisions. And I want the biopsy. I want to know as soon as possible what we're dealing with."

Leo and the doctor nodded in agreement. Two days later, Barbara went in for the biopsy. Her husband, mother, and two cousins went with her to the surgery. When Barbara awoke from the anesthesia, everyone was staring at her. Then, one by one, they left without saying a word until Leo was the only one left. He looked Barbara in the eye and said, "It is breast cancer. And you have to have it removed."

Barbara became hysterical. "Am I going to live? Am I going to live?" she shrieked. When he heard those words, Leo broke down and cried.

Then the doctor came in and looked at Barbara as though he didn't know what to say. The words "breast cancer" kept reverberating in her mind, echoing.

"Am I going to live?" she asked again, in a slow, even tone.

"I am going to do everything in my power so you do live," said the surgeon.

"I don't want to die," she whispered.

Leo told Lacey and Brooke, very simply, while Barbara watched. "Your mom is very sick," said Leo. "She's going to have to go to the hospital for a few days, so the doctors can make her better."

"Will she get better?" asked Lacey.

Leo nodded. He looked at Brooke, who didn't say a word.

"Are we still gonna have my birthday party?" Lacey asked.

"Of course," said Leo.

Lacey's party was at Chuck E. Cheese. She and her friends had a great time eating pizza, climbing through the tunnels, riding the bucking cars, and playing ball toss. Barbara moved slowly around the noisy, cavernous, neon-lit room, very aware of the cuplike device protecting her biopsy incision site. It was the most emotional party she could remember. She would glance down at her chest and feel a mixture of anger and fear. Then she'd look over as Brooke helped Lacey climb out of the ball pit, and a sense of relief and pride would wash over her. I'm so glad I'm here, she thought.

Before she went in for her mastectomy, Barbara told her supervisor about her diagnosis, explaining that she would have to take disability leave for a while. Having to say her diagnosis out loud, to someone other than her family, made it more real. And more scary. She kept thinking, I'm not going to come back. I'm going to die.

Barbara was very nervous about the surgery. She was very angry at God. "Why is this happening to me?" she demanded. "I thought you were supposed to watch out for good people!" Then she started to wonder: What kind of a person am I to have something so devastating happen?

Leo and her mother accompanied Barbara to the hospital. When she awoke, she felt a little nauseated, but she was just glad to wake up. She stayed in the hospital for five days, until both drains from her arms were removed. Leo came to visit her every day and even washed her hair, to the astonishment of the nurses.

Barbara avoided looking at her chest while she was in the hospital. She didn't want to see the blank spot and scar where her breast used to be. But once she got home, she had no choice. Now there were no nurses to change the bandages and clean the surgical site. Leo helped take care of the wound, but Barbara couldn't avoid seeing the scar. "It wasn't as bad as I had imagined it," Barbara said. "I think that was a big step for me, though, just looking at the scar."

Bearing the Burden

Barbara was terrified by chemo. The surgeon reassured her that she wouldn't lose all her hair. That thought made her feel much better. Her oncologist, on the other hand, wasn't exactly upbeat. At her first consultation, he told her, "You've been put on a very aggressive chemotherapy regimen, which will very probably make you really sick. In two weeks, you will lose all your facial hair, all the hair on your head."

Barbara became hysterical and started shouting. "First, they took my breast—they took my womanhood. And now they're going to take something else?" She tugged at the straight, light brown hair that hung past her shoulders. "Now everyone will know," she wailed.

Her oncologist added, "You should know that you won't be able to keep working during treatment."

Barbara and Leo left the office, even more distraught than before. "I know I can get disability, so we can handle my not working. But I'm having a really hard time coming to terms with losing all my hair," she told Leo.

Two days later, Barbara got another call to come back to the oncologist. This time, the news was good.

"Your lymph nodes came back negative," the oncologist said. "So the cancer hasn't spread." Barbara allowed herself a small smile. "I took your case back to the tumor board and they agreed to use a less aggressive treatment, since there's no lymph-node involvement." Barbara let out the breath she didn't realize she'd been holding. "You probably won't lose all your hair, though there will be some thinning."

This is a good day, Barbara thought. With no lymph node involvement, with no metastasis, I can beat this thing. I caught it early, she thought. I can do it.

Typically, Barbara received chemotherapy on a Friday, then went home, crawled into bed, and tried to sleep through the worst of it. Within two weeks, as predicted, her hair started falling out. She would brush her hair and after two strokes, the brush would be full of long, brown strands of hair. But also as predicted, she didn't lose all of it. She was grateful she had such thick hair. Rather than going totally bald or having large hairless patches, she simply had very thin hair.

The physical scarring wasn't as bad as Barbara had feared, but it left a mark on her emotions that was harder to handle. She felt like such a burden on her husband and children. Not only was she having a hard time holding up her end of the relationship—working and taking care of the kids and the house—but she couldn't even take care of herself anymore. She felt miserably sick and very sad. She just didn't want to live anymore.

Lacey had few questions for her parents. She would ask Barbara, "You okay, Mommy?" But she wasn't ready for much information. After Barbara's second hospitalization during treatment, Lacey became very clingy toward Barbara and didn't want to leave her sight. It got to the point where Lacey was afraid to go to school for fear her mother wouldn't be there when she got home.

At eight, Brooke was another story entirely. She wasn't ready for a lot of information either, but she responded to her mother's illness with intense anger. She resented that the family couldn't do all the activities they typically did, especially on chemo weekends. "Mommy's always sick, she's always sick," Brooke complained. "We never go to the movies or to the beach anymore. We never go roller-skating or bowling."

Barbara didn't understand Brooke's anger and was very hurt by it. She explained the situation to her doctor, who suggested that Barbara try to see things from an eight-year-old's perspective. "Eight-year-olds think the whole world revolves around them," he said. "She's not trying to hurt your feelings; she just wants her old life back."

Getting Through Each Day

To try to keep her mind off chemo and cancer, Barbara decided to do home day care, taking care of a cousin's infant. Since babies demand here-and-now attention, it was good therapy for Barbara. "It helps me spiritually and mentally," she explained.

Barbara also got lots of support from family, including her younger sister, Dawn, who helped Barbara out with the girls and the house while Leo was working.

For his part, Leo did everything in his power to help Barbara. He worked, watched the girls when he was off, and took on as much of the housework as he had time for. He did this while coping with a lot of frightening thoughts of his own. Leo worried about Barbara, about her treatment and her prognosis. He worried about the day-to-day logistics: working and taking care of his wife and daughters. He worried about the possibility of becoming a single parent, about raising two girls on his own. And he felt compelled to keep his spirits up, for the sakes of Barbara, Brooke, and Lacey.

Leo and Barbara would joke about it, guessing at what kind of woman Leo would choose if he remarried. "This has made us a lot stronger," said Barbara.

Barbara started going to a support group right after she was diagnosed. She thought it would be helpful to see other women experiencing the same problems. But she quickly stopped after four or five visits. She found the support group made her even more depressed. No one in the group really understood Barbara's situation. The youngest person she knew, the woman who had come to her hospital room as a Reach for Recovery volunteer, was a lot older than Barbara. "No one knew what I had to handle—what trouble signs I should look for in my daughters, how much or how little to tell them about my illness, how I worried about my sexuality and my husband. They were just so much older than me."

Barbara became very depressed while she was getting chemotherapy. She kept thinking that Leo couldn't possibly find her attractive. She didn't feel sexual; how could he find her appealing? "I didn't marry you for your breasts," Leo told her. She was lying in bed, feeling like she wanted to die. "I don't want to live anymore," she told Leo. "I wish I'd just die and then I wouldn't be a bother to you and the kids."

"You have two girls and you have me," he said. "There's nothing more I can give you. If that's not good enough for you to want to live, there's nothing I can do."

Barbara thought, if my husband can accept me, if he can find me sexy, I should be able to accept myself too. I should stop wallowing in self-pity.

However, her depression deepened when her doctors told her it wasn't a good idea for her to have any more children.

"The surgeon doesn't want me getting pregnant again," she told Leo. "And the oncologist says I *could* do it, but I should wait five years."

"I don't know about that," said Leo. "We are very lucky with Brooke and Lacey. Maybe we shouldn't take the chance of you getting pregnant again."

"But you always wanted a little boy to carry on your name," Barbara reminded him.

Much as he wanted a child to pass on his name, Leo had no trouble with the idea that Barbara shouldn't get pregnant again. To settle matters once and for all, Leo got a vasectomy. "Maybe I can convince the girls to stick with their maiden name," he told Barbara with a wink.

Reconstructing Herself

After she finished treatment, Barbara's oncologist brought up the question of reconstruction. "I'm not having any more surgery," Barbara said, remembering how uncomfortable she was after the mastectomy. "Besides, my surgeon said I shouldn't have reconstruction because I'm too big."

The oncologist wouldn't hear any of this. "First of all," he said, "You're young, you're only twenty-six years old. Second of all, you're *not* too big."

"I'm just not going to have any more surgery," Barbara decided, and had herself fitted with a prosthesis. The prosthesis worked fine during the day. She could wear a bra again, she could fit into all her shirts, and she felt balanced when she walked around.

But every morning as she dressed and every night as she undressed, Barbara was reminded that she was a cancer victim. She looked down at her long incision and mourned all over again. There wasn't a day she didn't think about having breast cancer. Grieving and grieving. She wasn't sure she could keep looking at it. But what was her alternative?

Barbara wanted to feel whole again, to be done with the prosthesis, and to avoid being confronted daily with her missing breast. So after a year of living with the prosthesis, Barbara decided to have reconstructive surgery. She was adamant that she didn't want anything foreign in her body. She wanted to use her own body tissue, so she opted for a TRAM flap procedure, which uses stomach tissue to reconstruct a breast mound. The surgery went well, and Barbara suffered no side effects.

"Look at this!" Barbara told Leo, "I can put on a bra and feel normal. I don't have to look down at a flat chest with a scar," she said, touching her left side. "It's the greatest feeling in the world. I'm not a cancer victim anymore. When I go to the beach, I can wear a bikini top and shorts. The scar will fade. Oh, it's just so wonderful to be able to fill out a bra."

"I've always thought you were beautiful," Leo said.

Barbara was realizing how glad she was to have two breasts. She decided to reduce the right breast, so they would both be the size she'd always wanted. She had been adamantly opposed to surgery, but she survived the reconstruction and saw what a positive change it had made in her life. Breast reduction, she believed, would do the same.

⋙⟐⟐

When Barbara finished reconstruction, she went back to the plastic surgeon for her six-week checkup. She was in a great mood. "I'm matching, I'm all healed, I'm good to go," she told him. Then the surgeon's serious look registered. "Oh my God. What now?"

"You have precancer in your right breast."

"I can't have precancer. I can*not* go through chemo again. I'm just twenty-seven years old. I just can't do it again."

"You have precancerous cells," he continued. "You don't have to have chemotherapy, you don't have cancer. But whether you choose to have a mastectomy or not is up to you. It's just a matter of waiting until it turns into cancer. It could be next week, it could be when you're thirty. We just don't know."

Barbara and Leo talked it over. "I'm scared," Barbara said.

"I agree. It feels like a time bomb. Have the mastectomy."

"Will you still want me?" asked Barbara, feeling like damaged goods. Leo just leaned over and gave her a big bear hug.

She opted for a mastectomy with immediate reconstruction. But she was told she could not have another TRAM flap operation. Her options were an eight-hour surgery using her back muscles or an implant, which would involve a series of minor surgeries. She chose a saline implant, feeling she'd already been through enough major operations.

Speaking to Congress

The plastic surgeon explained to Barbara that Congress was working to ban breast implants because of their potential health risks. Barbara was appalled; what would she have done, what about other women who had no other reconstruction choices? Her surgeon told her that he was going to Washington, D.C. to speak with Congress about the bill and encouraged her to come along with him. "You're so young, you'd be a good spokesperson," he explained.

So Barbara flew to Washington with her plastic surgeon and testified before Congress on the necessity for keeping breast implants available to women. The surgeon showed before and after pictures of Barbara's reconstruction—just the chest area, not her face.

"I didn't care. If that's what it takes to get the message across, then it's all right," said Barbara. "We gave Congress many reasons why they shouldn't ban breast implants. For one, some young girls don't develop breasts and for them, a breast implant is the only option they have for breast enhancement. It's the same for women who've been through breast cancer, who've had a mastectomy. If this is the only alternative they have, it's just not right to take it away," Barbara explained. She doesn't want women to go through the sadness she felt with her prosthesis if there was an alternative. She hopes her testimony helped make breast implants possible for other women.

"If it were your body, you'd want the choice, the option to make your own decision."

Role-Model Mom

Barbara started to think about what she wanted to do with the rest of her life. It was important to her that she set a good example for her children. She wanted them to see that she could plan her future—a future with them. That the breast cancer was something she'd overcome, and she wasn't going to give up. She completed her high school education and received her diploma, then enrolled in a few courses, including medical transcriptions, at the University of Southern Maine. It was hectic, juggling her child-care work, family, classes, and homework. She was hired in a surgical office near their home. She now feels as though she is making a contribution and doing work that is more interesting than factory shift work. And she is a good role model for her children: school is very important—and you're never too old to go back.

As Brooke grew older and entered high school, she became more comfortable discussing breast cancer with her parents. She wrote a paper on the disease for school and that seemed to open the door for discussions about Barbara's illness. Barbara was relieved; she'd been worried about Brooke's reluctance to talk.

Brooke also showed that she had been thinking about her mother all along. One day, Brooke's teacher sent home a sealed envelope addressed to Barbara. When she opened it up, Barbara gasped. Inside the envelope was an essay called "My Mother, My Hero." Brooke had written about Barbara, about how she dealt with breast cancer, went back to school, testified before Congress, and was a great role model for her girls.

Making Their Own Choices

Barbara continues to worry about the health of her daughters. Because of her diagnosis, both Brooke and Lacey are already at heightened risk for breast cancer. So Barbara wants to make sure that they don't add any other risk factors.

When Brooke turned seventeen, she began smoking cigarettes. Both Barbara and Leo were terrified of what it might mean for her health. And neither knew how to discourage her, since almost a decade of warnings clearly hadn't worked.

"You are responsible for the choices you make in life," said Barbara. "But I am going to have a hard time later on if you get breast cancer and you're sitting there smoking a cigarette. I mean, it's going to be hard to find compassion when you're taking that into your own hands," she told her daughter.

"But it's my decision," Brooke said. "You're just exaggerating, just harassing me."

"You have bronchitis," Barbara pointed out. "If you're going to continue to smoke, if you're going to make that decision, you're going to have to bear some of the consequences of the decision. You're going to have to shell out those co-pays for your doctor visits yourself."

The combination of cajoling and co-pays worked; Brooke quit smoking.

Barbara has also changed her outlook on life. "Before I had breast cancer, I felt like a day was just a day. I did things because I was supposed to, because it was expected," she told Leo. "I mean, I loved you, I loved Brooke and Lacey, but it felt a little routine, a little expected. Now I don't take anything for granted at all. I feel like my life is what I make it and if I want something, it's no one else's responsibility but mine to make changes in my life and to set goals for myself. And I've learned not to take things so much to heart. Every day is a good day. I'm really learning to let things go."

Barbara now does accounting work at a medical laboratory. She and Leo just celebrated their twentieth anniversary, and Brooke and Lacey are both in college. Barbara recently experienced some problems with her breast implant. After discussion with her surgeon, she has decided to undergo surgery to remove the implant and reconstruct her breast using her own tissue. She remains cancer free.

□ □ □

Children's reactions to a mother with breast cancer run the gamut. In general, younger children focus on more concrete concerns, whereas older children may be more reluctant to bring up the subject. Experts recommend addressing questions about breast cancer much the way you approach the dreaded "birds and bees" conversations. As with sex, experts recommend responding only to the questions asked, but answering them as openly and fully as possible. This approach should alleviate the fear and anxiety that children often feel when their mother is facing a life-threatening illness. Depending on the child, it may be upsetting to visit the hospital; some children do better with phone calls, so they don't have to see the fatigue and bandages.

Barbara's daughters were older when their mother became ill. As a result, they didn't ask questions explicitly so much as respond with fear about their mother's well-being and anger at the situation. They also addressed, albeit more obliquely, issues of cancer risk, when Brooke began to smoke.

When children raise issues obliquely, it can be harder to respond directly. But sometimes the direct approach is the only way. It is important that children understand what is going on with their mother, within their own emotional and intellectual limitations. Getting a handle on the situation can help them feel safer.

WHAT IF I HAVE THE BREAST CANCER GENE?

✺⟨⟩ Paulette, 25: Living with Uncertainty

PAULETTE PROGRESSED FROM FIFTEEN TO TWENTY-FIVE repetitions of each move. Always a slender woman, she focused on toning her biceps and triceps. She lifted twenty-pound weights with ease and smiled when she remembered the challenge that six pounds had presented when she first joined the gym. As her arms and legs grew stronger and her muscles more defined, Paulette had no inkling that her genetic structure was doing harm to the rest of her body.

She started coming to the gym because she knew no one in town. Married for a year and a half, Paulette and Jim moved seven hours south of their home to rural Jefferson, Georgia. They selected that location because they enjoyed country living. Jim commuted an hour west to a software company in Atlanta and Paulette drove twenty minutes east to her administrative assistant position in the college town of Athens. Since Jim spent so much time commuting, Paulette was alone a lot. She decided to turn extra time to her advantage and, at the same time, shed those few extra pounds. She could go from work to the gym and still beat her husband home.

The exercise was working. She'd toned up and her muscles were becoming well-defined. But so was a lump on her left breast. And the area was sore a lot.

⟳

Paulette didn't worry too much. After all, she'd had lumps in her breasts off and on while she was growing up, and they all went away with her menstrual cycle. Plus, she'd seen a physician's assistant through her HMO about the current lump just the previous September.

Paulette remembered feeling the muscles in her neck tighten as the physician's assistant picked up a tiny needle and anesthetized the skin around the lump. Her back had clenched as the physician's assistant selected a larger needle, attached the syringe, and guided it into the lump in Paulette's breast. She watched as the syringe did *not* fill up with fluid.

"It's not aspirating," the physician's assistant said in an even tone. "You're healthy and you're only twenty-five. You're too.young to have anything to worry about." She patted Paulette on the back and nudged her out the door. Paulette felt brushed off.

As the lump became more defined and more painful almost six months later, Paulette decided it was time to have it checked out again. When she called the HMO in March, she was more insistent and received a referral to a surgeon, who had her come to the hospital for a biopsy.

Jim was upbeat on the way to the hospital. He was certain Paulette would be fine. But she was scared. Call it intuition or sheer terror, but she was convinced there was something wrong with her breast. And she was worried about the care she would receive from an HMO that had dismissed her so easily before. As they prepped her for the biopsy surgery, Paulette stared at Jim's optimistic face, wishing she felt as he did. As soon as Paulette came out of the anesthetic, she heard the results: It was a tumor, and it was malignant.

Several days later, she got more detailed test results. The doctor called to say that the cancer had already spread throughout her breast ducts and that it would likely grow very aggressively. Paulette was stunned and in shock.

Her mother had a difficult time with the diagnosis. "She's convinced that it's her fault, somehow," Paulette said to Jim. "She likes to be a martyr."

"I don't understand," Jim said, always the calm, steady one. "There's no breast cancer at all on her side of the family."

Paulette nodded.

When Paulette called her father, however, she learned that while there was no cancer on her *mother's* side, there was a great deal of breast cancer on her father's side of the family. Her paternal grandmother died of breast cancer at the age of twenty-eight. All four of her father's sisters had had the disease: Anna died at age thirty-three, Harriet died in her late thirties, Barbara survived breast cancer but later succumbed to colon cancer, and Geraldine had breast cancer in her late twenties and was currently a twenty-five-year survivor. Harriet's two daughters, Tina and Toni, both developed breast cancer in their thirties, years before Paulette's diagnosis; Toni had died from the disease; Tina was still alive. Shortly after Paulette was first diagnosed, Geraldine's daughter Julie was also diagnosed with breast cancer, making her the eighth woman in the family to contract the disease, all well before the age of menopause.

Paying for Medical Care

As a result of the surgery, Paulette developed a hematoma—an internal blood blister—in her breast, which got infected and grew to the size of a grapefruit.

"It's huge," Paulette said. "And it hurts *so* much."

"I don't know about this HMO," Jim responded.

"I want a second opinion," Paulette said firmly. "I want to go to a reputable cancer center, even if it means going out of the HMO network."

"That would be very expensive," said Jim. "It could be around a thousand dollars for each chemo treatment." He rubbed his chin. "We'll just have to figure something out." Paulette could practically see cogs turning in his brain as his eyebrows grew into a single shaggy line.

"We'll have to take out a second loan on your Toyota."

"But we just paid it off." Paulette was amazed; Jim was usually so careful with money.

"You need a doctor who knows what he's doing," Jim replied.

⋇⟡⋇

Paulette was scared and she turned to Jeanette, her older sister, nine years her senior. Jeanette had always been a surrogate mother to Paulette. Jeanette arranged for Paulette to have a consultation at a major cancer center in North Carolina. Paulette moved up to stay with her sister in Lumberton, North Carolina, about ninety miles south of the medical center. Together, they hit the library, questioned friends and family members, and deciphered the information about Paulette's condition and about breast cancer in general. Jeanette took copious notes in a small notebook she bought specifically for that purpose. They created lists of questions, went to the doctor appointments, and kept track of the answers.

The first thing the doctor at the cancer center did was to aspirate the hematoma. During the two weeks it took for her chest to heal, Paulette went home to Jim in Georgia.

"Glad to have you back," Jim said, giving her a big hug.

But despite the warm welcome, Jim wasn't comfortable talking about breast cancer. He was scared he was going to lose his wife. He had watched his father die of lung cancer just a few years earlier. Throughout Paulette's diagnosis and treatment, Jim told only one friend about what was going on, a friend whose wife also had cancer. He just didn't know how to deal with his feelings.

Sisterly Compassion

When it was time to set up a treatment plan, Paulette headed back to North Carolina. Jim was worried about her, but looked relieved that she didn't ask him to go.

She went with Jeanette to speak with the surgeon and oncologist. The oncologist laid out her options: lumpectomy with radiation and possible chemotherapy. Or a mastectomy and chemo for sure.

"It looks like my only real option is a mastectomy," Paulette told the surgeon the next morning. "I want this over and done with."

Speaking to Jim on the phone that evening, Paulette said, "I just want to get rid of it. I'm not that attached to my breast at this point."

"That seems like the safest choice," Jim said without hesitation. "We don't want to go through this again." Then he added, "You know, I don't think I could do this as well as you're doing it." Paulette felt very reassured; she knew how hard it was for Jim to talk about his feelings.

Jeanette took Paulette to the hospital and offered to stay with her for all five days. Jim drove up from Georgia for the last two days and drove her back home.

Chemotherapy Collaboration

Paulette and Jim realized that they would not be able to afford to pay for her chemotherapy outside Paulette's HMO. But Paulette devised a plan: She asked the HMO oncologist to write up a chemotherapy protocol. She then asked the cancer center in North Carolina to take a look at it. To the couple's delight, the cancer center physicians agreed with the HMO protocol, so Paulette would be able to stay home in Georgia for treatment. Not only did it save them a bundle of money, but it meant that they could be together during this part of her treatment.

Paulette received chemo for six months. She scheduled her treatments to have minimum effect on her job. Every Friday, she left work at 2:30 and drove home to meet Jim, who took her to Atlanta for her 4:00 appointment. She sensed some resentment from her supervisor, but the other administrative assistants seemed understanding about her illness.

One Monday, after Paulette had been receiving chemo for several weeks, she went to lunch with a friend from work. "You know, your boss resents that you leave early on Friday, even though you don't take lunch," her friend confided. "She spends Friday afternoons telling everybody what a lousy job you do, how you never meet your deadlines, and how you leave early twice a month."

Paulette was livid. "Let me get this straight: I'm getting treatment for a life-threatening disease and she's bad-mouthing me because I miss two hours of work on a Friday? Maybe she wants to spend *her* weekends throwing up?"

Paulette was so upset that she apologized to her friend and left the restaurant. She raced out the door, slammed her way into her car, and called Jim.

"I can't believe what's going on. I just don't want to work there, I can't show my face there anymore," she sobbed into the phone.

"If you're that unhappy," he said sympathetically, "just quit. It isn't worth it."

At 5:00, when Paulette left the office, she cleaned out her desk, deposited her key in an envelope, and slid it under the door with a letter of resignation. Effective immediately.

⟡

Paulette needed to talk to someone who understood what it felt like to have a life-threatening disease. She tried a Reach for Recovery support group, but felt very uncomfortable. All the other women had grown children and most had grandchildren. By contrast, Paulette was twenty-five. All she had in common with the rest of the group was cancer. Fortunately, through her doctor's office, she met three other women with breast cancer who were around her age. The four young women got together periodically, usually for dinner in a restaurant, to trade stories and ask advice. They all appreciated knowing women their own age who were in breast cancer treatment. Paulette enjoyed talking to people who really knew what it was like.

Ultimately, however, two of the young women died; their cancers had spread beyond their breasts. Their deaths scared Paulette; breast cancer was frightening, but when it spread, it became completely terrifying.

Thinking Reconstruction

When she had her mastectomy, Paulette wasn't sure she wanted to reconstruct her breast. She didn't want any more surgery; she felt the doctors had done enough to her body. The only option presented to her at that point was immediate reconstruction with an implant, which was not much of an option in her eyes.

But the prosthesis became a constant reminder. Finally, two years after the diagnosis, Paulette felt ready.

But she wanted it to be as safe a procedure as possible. That meant no implants, Paulette decided. She had the rest of her life to think about. And she didn't want to have problems down the line because of implants. That left Paulette with the option of more complicated surgeries, most of which would involve moving fat from one part of her body to her chest.

She sat in her plastic surgeon's office and went through the options. "At five-foot-nine and one hundred and twenty-five pounds, you just don't have the stomach for a TRAM flap surgery," he said. "And a latissimus flap would require an implant."

"That's out of the question," Paulette responded quickly. She'd had enough of life-threatening conditions; she wanted a safe option, if there was one. If not, well, she'd lived with a prosthesis this long. A smile spread across her face. "My ass is so big, can't you use that?"

The doctor laughed. "As a matter of fact, we *could* do a gluteal free flap," he suggested.

That's what Paulette chose to do. The surgeon transferred tissue from her buttocks, including skin, fat, and gluteus muscle, and using microsurgery, attached the flap and formed a new breast.

≈

Jeanette tracked the study of the genetics of breast cancer in the news. She called her doctor to ask if there was a study that her family could get involved in. She reminded him how many of her relatives had developed breast cancer premenopausally. The researchers were immediately interested and began taking medical histories and blood samples from everyone except her brother, who assiduously avoided the researchers. He seemed to have convinced himself that breast cancer was passed only through women, and he did not intend to have children. Jeanette, who had long worried about her lumpy breasts, didn't have the gene. But Paulette's tests came back positive.

Going to see the oncologist every six months for a battery of examinations was starting to wear on Paulette. She asked her oncologist to put her on an annual checkup schedule. He promised her he would after it had been five years from her diagnosis.

Meanwhile, Jim was worrying about the cancer gene, called BRCA1, and began thinking prevention. "Have you considered a prophylactic mastectomy?" he asked. "Do you think they should remove your right breast so it can't develop cancer?"

Paulette was surprised by his suggestion. Other than finances and logistics, this was the first time Jim had made a suggestion about the treatment of her disease; he'd mostly just followed her lead. "That's an interesting idea. I sure don't know what I'd do if they found cancer again. But it seems so radical, don't you think?"

"I don't know about the medical part," Jim continued slowly. Paulette knew he'd thought a lot about this suggestion—he wasn't an "off-the-cuff" kind of guy. "But I don't think they've been proactive enough, and I don't want to go through this again. Could you ask your oncologist what he thinks?" Paulette agreed to ask.

"It's too aggressive," the oncologist said. "Your mammograms and blood work have all been normal. And most recurrences happen in the first two years; you've been fine for three years. We're monitoring you closely. I really don't think it's necessary."

Quietly, Paulette agreed. She didn't regret her mastectomy; it made sense medically. But she felt like part of her was missing now, the reconstructed breast just didn't seem real. She didn't want to lose her one remaining breast unless she absolutely *had* to.

Moving On

That fall, Paulette and Jim were ready to leave town. They had bought a piece of land just outside Chapel Hill, North Carolina, before they had gotten married. They told each other they were holding onto the land because they hadn't gotten a good enough offer to sell it, but Paulette knew they'd always hoped to move back. Plus, the experience with breast cancer made the couple lonely; they missed their family and friends. Jim applied for a position as a software engineer in Research Triangle Park, near Chapel Hill. He was offered the position and accepted it. Paulette was thrilled; she had no job and few friends to tie her to Georgia. She wondered whether they should try to have a child once they got settled. But they agreed to wait.

They decided to build a house on the parcel of land that they owned. A friend warned Paulette that building a house could be a true test of a marriage. Paulette just laughed. "We've been though breast cancer; building a house should be easy."

Events moved with surprising speed. Shortly after the move, Paulette received a job offer with the local university. It was an administrative position, similar to what she had been doing in Athens. The day after she accepted the position, three years after she finished treatment, she started to feel extremely tired and a little queasy. "I can't be pregnant," Paulette told herself. "We're not even trying." After a few more days of symptoms, Paulette took a home pregnancy test, with Jim at her side. Before she looked at the paper, she closed her eyes for a moment, hoping for a negative result. She opened her eyes and looked at Jim. Together, they stared at the thin blue line. She kept thinking that any child she had would have a fifty/fifty chance of having the breast cancer gene. She was nervous, but decided to hope for the best; after all, even having the gene doesn't necessarily mean having cancer. She didn't worry about pregnancy affecting her chances of recurrence because her cancer was estrogen-receptor-negative, so it was unclear that increasing hormones would have any effect.

꽃೧Ͼ

Claire was born in July 1993. When her daughter was ten months old, Paulette had her four-year checkup: a perfectly normal mammogram. The following September, Paulette thought she felt a lump in her right breast. It was just before her period, so she convinced herself that it was due to normal hormonal fluctuations. Then she went in for her six-month checkup; at this point, she was four and a half years out from her initial diagnosis.

The nurse examined her breast and kept returning to the same spot, with a furrow between her eyebrows. "You really should get this checked out, just to be safe," she said and sent Paulette down to the radiology department. There she received repeated mammograms, which was alarming because the last time this had happened, Paulette was diagnosed with breast cancer. Then the technician said she would also need a sonogram. At that point, Paulette started to get agitated and began asking if there was something the matter with the machinery or whether they were checking out something suspicious on the tests. The technician ignored her questions, then said, "The radiologist wants to see you."

The doctor walked in. "Oh, I can see you're upset," she began.

"Of course I'm upset," Paulette said, trying not to raise her voice. Call it intuition or experience, but she knew what was ahead: a second cancer diagnosis, a second mastectomy. "You're not giving me any information. It's not like I haven't been here before." After radiology, she went to the surgeon, who aspirated some cells and confirmed the malignancy.

Once she scheduled the mastectomy, Paulette called her sister. "I guess the second diagnosis of breast cancer was probably inevitable," she said. "Even if they'd been more aggressive with chemo the first time, it wouldn't have helped. The outcome would have been the same," she sighed, "because I have the gene."

A Child's Questions

When Paulette felt well enough, shortly after she came home from the hospital after her second mastectomy, she took a bath with eighteen-month-old Claire, as she had done all the child's life.

"Where is it?" Claire asked in a whisper, pointing to Paulette's chest.

"The doctors took my breast off," Paulette said in as soothing a voice as she could muster. She didn't mention that the one breast Claire saw was a reconstruction. "They had to take it off to get rid of the cancer."

Claire just stared at her mother's uneven chest without a word. Paulette wished there was an easy way to explain the uncertainty without revealing the terror she felt. Sometimes it seemed like the hardest part about having breast cancer was telling Claire.

"The cancer made mommy very sick," Paulette continued. "But if mommy takes her medicine, she will get better."

"Mommy take medicine?" Claire asked. Paulette nodded.

She knew the chemotherapy would be much more aggressive this time around. It *had* to be. "You'd better kick my ass good," she told her oncologist, "because I'm not doing this again. I will not go through this again."

As she had feared, it took only two treatments for her hair to start falling out. One night, after Claire had gone to sleep, Paulette and Jim were sipping a beer and talking about her hair. "I don't want to wake up one morning with my hair all fallen out," she told him. "I want you to shave my head. Right now. I could just cut it short, but it's an issue of control. I want to be in control of my body, not the disease." She walked over to the kitchen, put a clean dishtowel around her neck, and sat down facing the wall. Jim picked up the clippers.

The next morning, Claire was confused. She kept looking at Paulette's head as if to say, "I know you had hair when I went to sleep last night." That night, in the bath, the questions came.

"Where is your hair?"

"You know mommy has cancer," Paulette began slowly. "Mommy takes medicine to make the cancer go away. The medicine makes mommy's hair fall out, but it makes me better."

For her second reconstructive surgery, Paulette chose a TRAM free flap. "I've gained a lot of weight," she told her sister. "Now it's not a problem to use the fat from my stomach."

She had a good rapport with her surgeon who, incidentally, had trained under her first plastic surgeon, which boded well. The surgery was scheduled for the day after the big college basketball game. "Are you going to stay up all night and watch the ball game?" Paulette half-joked with the doctor. "Because I don't want you drinking a whole lot of coffee tomorrow morning and being jittery when you operate on me."

Facing the Future Together

"Finding out about the cancer this time was much more frightening," Paulette told Jim. "Now I look at Claire and wonder how much of her life I'll see: Will I be around to see her graduate high school? Will I be around to see her get married? It may be a cliché, but it's my biggest fear."

"Are you going to have Claire tested for the BRCA1 gene?" Jeanette asked one night.

"They can't do the test until she's at least thirteen and they don't recommend it until she's old enough to make the decision herself, until she's about eighteen," Paulette said, sighing into the phone. "What good would it do? Would it change the way she lives her life?"

"I guess not," said Jeanette. "But I could see how some mothers might want to know about their daughters."

"People have control over some things," Paulette said. "You can control what you eat, how you vote. But some things, like breast cancer, are just handed to you." The phone was silent. "I figure there is some reason I got breast cancer," Paulette continued. "I don't know what the reason is, what I'm supposed to do. But, please, let me get it right this time. I know I need to help other people. And I hope that speaking at local high schools, counseling women in the hospital, and raising money through the Race for the Cure is enough."

Ox

When Paulette and Claire were taking a bath together after the second reconstruction, Claire began to ask more questions. "Did the doctor use a knife?"

"Yes, he did," Paulette said as she rubbed at Claire's knees with a washcloth.

"Was it a sharp knife?"

"Well, Claire, it didn't hurt," Paulette dropped the washcloth back into the soapy water. "I was asleep." Paulette wasn't sure how to reassure her daughter about surgery. Nor was she sure how to reassure herself. All she could do was to hope for a cure in her daughter's lifetime.

Paulette still lives in central North Carolina with her husband and preteen daughter. She is now fifteen years beyond her first breast cancer diagnosis and is doing well. She is very active in the Susan G. Komen Race for the Cure; Claire runs the race alongside her mother. It has become a bonding experience for them both. Claire has a few more years before she wants to be tested for the breast cancer gene.

□ □ □

The question of passing on the breast cancer gene doesn't arise for most women. As of 2003, two genes have been identified that bring an increased risk for developing breast and ovarian cancer. But the BRCA1 and BRCA2 genes account for approximately 5 to 10 percent of breast cancer cases. And having the gene doesn't mean you'll pass it on to your daughter; while Dawn has the gene, her daughter—much to her mother's delight—does not carry it.

However, one of the risk factors for breast cancer is having a mother or sister who has had the disease, even if no one in the family carries either the BRCA1 or the BRCA2 gene. This is an issue that many women face when they decide whether to have a child after battling the disease. Indeed, the quandary promoted Lanita to adopt. "I would never forgive myself if I had a girl and she ended up having breast cancer," she said. Similarly, Susan, who opted to give birth, says, "I hope and pray that I made the right decision for myself and for Diana."

⚬

Parenting can complicate the already challenging physical and emotional effects of breast cancer diagnosis and treatment for women of any age. But young women have particular concerns, as they are more likely to have young children at the time they are diagnosed, or not to have any yet. Whereas older women worry about how to tell their grown children, women ages forty and younger are more likely to hear questions about hospital stays and balding and complaints about decreased energy levels.

Women in their childbearing years are also more likely to be faced with questions of reproduction. Has chemotherapy rendered them infertile? If so, do they want to adopt? If they are able to have children, do they want to take on the risk to themselves and their children, especially daughters? And then, if they already have children or decide to have children after treatment, young women who have had breast cancer face questions about their own mortality. Both Paulette and Barbara wondered if they would be around to see their children graduate from high school. The answers vary based on health and life situation.

The flip side of these concerns is the revitalizing nature of having and raising children. Susan decided that she wanted a child, in part because she kept hearing women say that their family got them through the breast cancer experience.

Survivor Suggestions on Pregnancy, Children, and Family

☐ Explore fertility options early on, if that is a concern.

☐ Show the love you feel for members of your family. And let them show you. Accept, and ask for, help from parents and other family members.

☐ Take care of your support system; give them time and space to come to terms with the situation, the way they are doing for you.

☐ Remember that life goes on during breast cancer treatment, especially if you have kids.

☐ Trust in your children's strength.

☐ Give young children the information they request; answer their questions as they arise, but don't add more than they are ready to hear. You don't want to frighten them.

☐ Be prepared for different children to respond differently, even within the same family.

☐ Remember that children focus on themselves, so don't expect to receive the same level of sympathy from a child as you would from an adult.

☐ Try not to make major changes in your children's lives while they are dealing with you having breast cancer.

☐ Be vigilant about your children's health.

☐ If you have a breast cancer gene, learn everything you can about it. It does not mean, for instance, that you will get cancer, only that you have increased risk for the disease. Consider having your daughter tested. But it should be your daughter's decision.

☐ Friends and family should not keep secrets from you just because you are in treatment for breast cancer; sometimes the disease gives you additional insights. Also, it is important for you to feel a part of the family or friendship.

☐ If you don't want to discuss all the details over and over, set up a phone (or e-mail) tree; update one or two people and have them pass the news along. They can answer questions and help people figure out the best way to help and be supportive.

🎕 Chapter Five 🎕

Faith, Religion, and Spirituality

Barbara was very angry at God: "Why is this happening to me?
I thought you were supposed to watch out for good people!"

PEOPLE VARY IN THEIR FEELINGS toward a higher being, toward for-malized ritual, and toward a search for answers. And these meanings can change throughout one's lifetime, especially in response to a life-threatening disease such as breast cancer. Extreme circumstances—difficult choices, living with uncertainty, facing one's mortality—often lead people to discover the role of prayer and spirituality in their lives. Each of the women in this chapter encountered a crisis in her spiritual life when she came face-to-face with breast cancer.

Dana had always had a strong sense of herself as a Jew. She found Jewish ritual to be a source of strength and worked with her rabbi to create a ceremony to say "goodbye" to one breast and a second cere-mony before her second mastectomy.

Robin turned to faith not so much for specific answers but as a way to pose questions. She sees the very process of rethinking her life and priorities in the face of breast cancer as a spiritual undertaking. Her feeling about religion or faith is "less about how it helps—the way aspirin can help a headache—than how it may be a thread in our daily lives that takes on a more potent role under certain conditions."

Breast cancer brought Dawn to a new and stronger personal relationship with religion. She found greater meaning as a born-again Christian than as a Catholic, and her children followed in her footsteps. (Her husband, conversely, began to question religion after Dawn's diagnosis and stopped attending church altogether.)

Through emotional, ritual, and philosophical questions, women often find faith to be an integral part of rebuilding and directing their lives after breast cancer.

HOW CAN RITUAL HELP ME?

✺ Dana, 26: Feeling Blessed

DANA DIDN'T REALLY KNOW STEPHEN, her new roommate, well enough to make a request like this. She and her friend Jill and Jill's friend Stephen had moved into the Eastside Milwaukee apartment only a month earlier and, shortly after their moving-in party, Jill left for California to do a medical residency, leaving two virtual strangers sharing a three-bedroom apartment.

Dana had ignored the lump for a week, chalking it up to her bony physique and menstrual changes. Tonight she felt the lump again, and this time she couldn't dismiss it so easily. She had to check it out, and Stephen was, after all, well on his way to being a doctor. Perhaps he could be helpful, possibly even reassuring. His door was closed; he was probably asleep. But Dana decided that she felt more nervous about the lump than guilty over possibly waking her roommate. Dana knocked on his bedroom door. She heard his muffled "Come in," and entered his room.

"Stephen, I hate to bother you, but will you feel my breast? I think I feel a lump." Dana spoke rapid-fire, wanting to get this over as quickly as possible. "Could you tell me what you think?"

Stephen reached his arm out from under the blanket, one eye open, and tried to locate the spot. "This feels significant," he said, stopping at the lump she had found. He tried to be comforting and suggested that Dana try to get some sleep. As she left the room, Dana began to cry. She prayed to God that this was nothing, that Stephen was wrong.

The next morning, Dana realized she had to cancel her dinner date with Adam, a friend of Jill's she had met at their apartment-warming party.

She called him and explained, "I really would like to have dinner with you. I don't want you to think I'm blowing you off, so let me tell you what's going on," Dana began, direct as ever. "I found a lump on my left breast and I have to get it checked out."

That weekend, Dana was a bridesmaid in the wedding of one of her closest friends. Dana didn't want to ruin her friend's special day. Her parents, Arlene and Howard, and one other couple were the only people at the wedding aware of the lump.

Dana's parents went with her to see her oncologist that Monday morning. The doctor did a needle biopsy on Tuesday. By Wednesday, the results were back: lots of normal cells and just a few abnormal ones. Dana was relieved; maybe it was going to be all right. Because the results weren't conclusive, the doctor scheduled an "open," or more extensive, biopsy for Thursday.

Not the First Time

Even before she found the lump in her breast, Dana was already a cancer survivor. Her first experience with cancer began when she was nineteen, a sophomore at the University of Wisconsin–Madison. She was home in Milwaukee for spring break. During her routine annual physical, the internist found a lump on her neck.

Dana nicknamed the lump "Moe the Mass."

"Moe's got to go," she told her friends, and was scheduled for surgery to remove the lump.

Dana's family was with her in the recovery room when the surgeon came in to speak with them. Lab reports done on the tumor revealed that Dana had Hodgkin's disease, he told them. But it could be cured with radiation therapy. He set an appointment for Dana with an oncologist.

Dana and her oncologist devised a plan: Shrink the tumor with chemotherapy, then follow with radiation therapy. Due to complications with the treatment, however, she ended up receiving more chemo than originally planned.

Chemotherapy and radiation completed, Dana went back to school in Madison, monitored closely by her doctors. At five years after treatment for Hodgkin's, Dana was considered "cured." But whenever Arlene said that, Dana balked. "I don't want you to use that word. It's not that I'm not in remission—I am. But not a day goes by that I don't worry about getting sick again."

Dana had periodic scares throughout her time at Madison. She would feel a lump under her arm or on her leg and immediately make an appointment with her oncologist and head to Milwaukee. She felt like a hypochondriac, but decided that she would rather feel secure in her health than worry about embarrassment.

❧

Now, as Dana and her parents drove to the breast surgeon's office for the open biopsy, Dana realized that she was upset. "I *asked* my oncologist if all the radiation I received for Hodgkin's disease could lead to more cancer and he was never straight with me," she complained. "And now I find out that it *can* increase the risk of breast cancer."

At this biopsy, the surgeon extracted a lump the size of two grapes and sent it off to the lab for testing. The results were back Saturday morning. It was breast cancer.

Dana was stunned. She called her oncologist at home to discuss the basics of treatment: surgery and chemotherapy.

God Gets the Message

When she heard the news, Dana quit her job as a pediatric social worker at a local hospital and moved back to her parents' home temporarily. Immediate family, extended family, friends, and friends of friends rallied around. "It was an amazing feeling to know that I could call on as many people as I needed. I felt like I could never really fall, that someone would always be there to catch me," Dana said.

She got phone calls from friends all around the country and from people she barely remembered, cards and flowers from people she had met only briefly in the hospital, all saying, "We're praying for you." Dana figured God had to get the message. As she told Arlene, "There are all these telephone calls to God and if God doesn't want to answer one, he's certainly going to get another. He's being bombarded."

Flowers arrived daily and filled every corner of the house. Dana jokingly greeted people at the door saying, "Welcome to my funeral parlor."

For her birthday in October, Dana's friends threw her a party. People drove from all over the Midwest and flew in from California just to see her. Dana was deeply touched by their efforts and wrote a long thank-you letter to Sheryl and Jon, the couple who had orchestrated the get-together. She wrote, in part:

> Since the diagnosis of breast cancer, I've been searching for a reason. And last night shed so much light on the bigger meaning. I've always considered myself lucky and extremely blessed, but it's people like you that make it so. I know the next months will be rough times, but the memories of the love, the feelings from this weekend, will get me through it. With all my heart, I thank you for a beautiful, wonderful evening and more importantly for a friendship and love that knows no boundaries.

Now that her diagnosis was certain, the next step was to determine the extent of the cancer, a process called staging the disease. Dana's cousin Jeffrey, a radiologist, told her, "You have the time to make an informed decision about your doctor and your treatment. The cancer has been in you for a while and you have a couple of weeks to make a decision."

"But I have *cancer*," Dana said. "I have to figure it out *now*."

"You can take three weeks to get different opinions and see what your treatment options are," Jeffrey reassured her.

Dana got opinions from several hospitals in Chicago and Milwaukee, each time meeting with an oncologist, a breast surgeon, a radiation oncologist, and a plastic surgeon.

She bought a spiral-bound notebook and began to collect information, with help from her parents, who attended every appointment. Dana made a point of reading all her reports and looking at all her films. She brought a list of questions to every appointment and wrote down the doctor's responses. "It's a terrible feeling to walk out of an appointment and then remember the most important question," she told her mother.

Dana began treatment with her original oncologist, the one who had treated her Hodgkin's disease when she was a teenager. Because the size (nine centimeters) and position (near the chest wall) of Dana's cancer indicated that Dana was in stage III breast cancer, the doctor decided to start with chemotherapy to shrink the tumor. He recommended she then have surgery to remove the tumor, followed by more chemotherapy treatment.

But Dana wasn't comfortable with him anymore. She found herself second-guessing every decision, mostly because he never acknowledged that the radiation treatment she received for Hodgkin's disease had increased her risk of breast cancer. After much thought, Dana decided to switch her care to the head of the oncology department at a nearby teaching hospital. While the doctor there was very busy and she would probably end up seeing a backup oncologist some of the time, she would be able to tap into the department chief's vast experience and take advantage of the hospital's state-of-the-art technology.

"I really appreciate everything you've done for me," Dana said as she looked at the oncologist who helped her through her first battle against cancer. "But I find I'm not trusting your decisions because of our history." She cried as she explained her decision to move her care from his office to the teaching hospital.

"It is really important to me that there are no hard feelings," she said at last.

"Dana," said the oncologist, holding out his hand, "I think of you as a daughter."

Though she knew chemo would be draining, Dana was eager to regain some of her independence. She moved back in with Jill and Stephen as she began five cycles of chemotherapy. Her mother took her to each treatment.

"I hate that color, I hate that bright red," she would say as the nurse approached her with the cancer-fighting drug injection.

"But why?" the nurse would say. "It's the color of love, it's passion."

"It's gross," Dana said, wincing every time.

Dana took some medication to boost her white blood cell count, but it made her bones and back ache. It seemed like she could actually feel her body working to reproduce the blood cells. She also took an anti-nauseant, which she described to friends and family as "my best friend."

In Search of Support

Despite the loving support she received from her family and friends, Dana began to realize that she needed to talk to *young* people—women her own age—who knew how it felt to hear the words, "You have breast cancer."

She chased down the Reach for Recovery volunteer who had called her and requested a face-to-face meeting. She talked to young people she saw in her oncologist's office. She would tell her mother, "I've got to go introduce myself. That person is young and she has cancer." And she put her name on every support group list she could find.

She tried one group, held in a dreary, dimly lit room. People were speaking softly and the discussion seemed to center around one severely depressed woman. Dana didn't find the group cathartic; she could almost hear a funereal chant in the background. She went two or three more times, but then decided that the group wasn't going to help her and stopped going.

"With my social work background, I know it's important to have a support group," Dana told her mother. So she tried another group, one geared to breast cancer survivors who had chosen reconstruction. She walked in, looked around the room, and felt like crying. About thirty breast cancer survivors were sitting in a circle of chairs, but Dana was the youngest by far. Many of the women could have been her mother or grandmother. She decided to stick it out and see how it went.

After about half an hour, during the questions and answer session that followed the more formal presentation, someone asked, "Aren't you Adam's friend?"

"Yes," Dana said.

"We work in the same office. We went out to lunch a couple of weeks ago because he was concerned about you and I was the only person he knew who'd had breast cancer."

Ten minutes later, a woman sitting across the room asked, "Are you Dana? Does your mother work at Jewish Community Day School?"

"Yes, that's me."

"I've heard all about you. My name is Felice."

Within the hour, Dana felt at home in the group. She was younger, true, but she felt connected with the group; these women had gone through similar experiences and were upbeat. "They were just eating up life," she told her mother that evening. She also tried—and stuck with—a second group of about a dozen breast cancer survivors; these two groups helped pull her through her illness.

Life Goes On

Dana had quit her clinical job, but she knew she didn't want to sit at home during treatment. So she called a woman at a college Hillel organization with whom she had once interviewed. She had really hit it off with the director of the on-campus Jewish center, but had turned down the position because she wanted a full-time job. Now, though, part-time was looking good. "Come in to the office, we'll talk," the woman said.

"Here's the situation," Dana began. "I'll be starting chemotherapy next week. I don't know how I'll be feeling. I don't know how many hours I can put in."

"Of course."

"It would have to be an open relationship. If it's not working for me, I would just stop. And if you find that I'm not giving you what you need, you would have to tell me that, too. We would have to agree that there would be no hard feelings."

The director leaned across the table to Dana and gave her a kiss. "Be well. I'll see you on Monday."

※

Dana kept busy during chemo. She worked five to ten hours a week at the Hillel center, went out with family and friends, took art classes at the local museum, and attended two support groups.

She also continued to date Adam, who was very supportive, often offering "Adam medicine"—companionship, a long talk, or a big bear hug—when she wasn't feeling well. But Dana didn't take their relationship seriously. It was a strange time to date; they were still getting to know each other, so she didn't feel she could share all of her feelings with him. She also didn't really have the energy to invest in a serious relationship. She just wanted to have fun, go dancing. Dana decided to break it off. She felt uncertain and scared, worried about sharing so much with Adam, and asking so much of him.

"I just don't think this is a good time for me. You're a really sweet man," she told him. "But the timing just isn't right. I'm scared about my surgery in January and I want to focus on getting ready."

Blessings in Healing Waters

Meanwhile, Dana was thinking about her mastectomy and doing everything she could to prepare herself emotionally for the operation. She practiced visualization and imagery work. She bought meditation tapes. She read about the psychology of breast cancer patients. She saw a psychologist and continued with her support groups. She tried to express her feelings through humor, laughter, and music, writing new lyrics to the Everly Brothers' song "Bye Bye Love," calling it "Bye Bye Tumor."

Dana read a lot and learned that spirituality was a great healing tool for many breast cancer survivors. Because Judaism had long been a source of strength for her, she decided to create her own ceremony to prepare for the mastectomy. She spoke with a rabbi in a large synagogue in Chicago, thinking a female rabbi would better understand her concerns. But she ended up working with the male rabbi at her local synagogue because—to her surprise—*he* was the one who validated all of her feelings.

The ceremony centered on the *mikveh*. In Jewish tradition, the mikveh is a natural body of water (usually a pool or a stream) where a person who has become ritually impure purifies him or herself by immersion. Mikvehs were common in biblical times; nowadays, many are bathhouses and are used most often by observant women after menstruation and people converting to Judaism or getting married. Before writing this ceremony, Dana had never been to a mikveh. She envisioned a dark room with a pool of cloudy water.

The rabbi explained that mikvehs are healing waters. He told her that they signal transitions, such as conversion or marriage. Dana worked hard at writing a ceremony, gathering material from a variety of Jewish and non-Jewish sources. "It's a bit of a hodgepodge," Dana told her mother, "with secular self-healing affirmation and ideas from

Reform and Conservative Judaism and the Bible." The rabbi worked with Dana to be certain that the ceremony followed all relevant Jewish laws.

When she arrived at the mikveh on the day of the ceremony, Dana was impressed by how bright, clean, and beautiful it was. With soothing pastel walls and a neat and clean appearance, the mikveh felt like a resort. I can see feeling pampered here, she thought.

Dana handed out the scripts to her mother, her cousin Patty, and her friends Sheryl and Becky, keeping one for herself. Then she disrobed and carefully lowered herself into the pool, under the gentle supervision of a woman from the mikveh.

Dana began, "Today I ask God for help in every way. God, speak through me, God, act through me. In my faith and trust and comfort and humility, I ask for the help of God that I so desperately need."

Dana's mother continued, "By the God of your parents who will help you. By Shaddai who will bless you with the blessings of the heavens and the blessings of the mysteries of creation, blessings of the breast and blessings of the womb."

"Be strong and of good courage," Sheryl quoted from the book of Joshua. "Fear not nor be afraid for the Lord thy God will not fail thee or forsake thee."

After comments from Patty and Becky, Dana recited a blessing, immersed herself in the mikveh water twice, said another blessing, and then immersed herself a third time.

"Eternal one who is my light, my salvation, whom shall I fear?" Sheryl recited. "God is my stronghold of my life, of whom shall I be afraid?"

Patty and Arlene read about the importance of God's unconditional love and hope, then Dana discussed the sympathy for suffering that she hopes to gain from her experience. She recited two more blessings: "*Baruch atta adonai rafeya holei amo yisrael*. I praise You, O God, the one Who heals the people of Israel. *Baruch atta adonai elohenu melekh haolam shehehiyanu vikiyemanu vihigiyanu lazman hazeh*. Blessed art Thou, O Lord our God, King of the universe, Who has kept us alive, and sustained us, and enabled us to reach this season." Dana immersed herself in the mikveh one final time.

After Becky, Sheryl, and Patty offered inspirational sayings, everyone expressed their wishes for Dana's health and for all who "suffer illness of body and mind."

Then Dana and all of the witnesses said a final blessing and sang the Shema, a prayer that celebrates the oneness of God.

Dana's mother placed her hands on Dana's head, saying, "May God bless you and protect you like Sarah, Rebecca, Rachel, and Leah. May the light of God shine upon you and God's grace be with you. May God be with you always and bring peace to you."

"Amen."

"The process of writing the ceremony was the most meaningful aspect for me," Dana told her mother, cousin, and friends after the ceremony. "Finding pieces that would be comforting, shaping them into a ceremony, asking people to participate—that was the special part."

Like Kojak, but with Lipstick

Dana had the mastectomy on her left side that January. She woke up from the anesthesia and was terrified to look down at her chest. She was certain her chest would be horribly ugly. In fact, she'd prepared her father for the worst, told him she might be crying for weeks on end.

But when she saw her chest, she said out loud, "It's not that bad. It's not ugly—it's just not there." She decided that it was a badge of honor to have her breast removed. She felt like a warrior. God forbid it should happen to anyone else, but *she* was going to be all right.

The surgery was a success: The margins were clean and no lymph nodes were affected. But she would never know whether the nodes had been fine or whether the first five cycles of chemo had simply eliminated the cancer.

Three more cycles of chemo followed. They were hard, much more difficult than the first five cycles; her body was worn out from treatment.

She knew she was going to lose her hair. She wasn't looking forward to it; she'd already lost it twice: once when she was treated for

Hodgkin's disease and again with her first round of chemotherapy treatment for breast cancer.

Dana and her younger brother Richie had made a pact that once her hair began to fall out, he would shave her head. They would make the loss of Dana's hair into a joke, a mini-party for brother and sister. One Sunday afternoon, about six weeks into treatment, Dana decided that it was time.

She stood looking into her bathroom mirror with a fluffy towel wrapped around her neck. Richie stood behind her, clippers in his right hand. His fiancée, Andrea, sat on the tub watching as Richie shaved one side.

Dana looked in the mirror and her mouth dropped open. She looked so...so...*bald*. "Richie," she said softly. "I think I have to do this myself."

He put the clippers down and kissed Dana's head.

Richie and Andrea stayed with Dana for several hours, comforting her. The next morning, Dana finished shaving the rest of her head. In the end, she liked the way it looked. Sort of Sinéad O'Connor-ish. Sort of cool. She couldn't wait to show her friends.

Sometimes she was ill, sometimes she felt okay, always she was bald. Every so often, she would get tired of wearing wigs and just put on bright lipstick and funky earrings and call it a day. "Let people stare at me. Who cares if I look like Kojak?" she told her friends.

Dana continued to get together with Adam casually, often in a group of friends. Then he got a new job as a branch manager for an electrical supply company and moved to Chicago. Dana went there several times to visit. And just when she thought it was safe—when Adam was living ninety miles away from Milwaukee—she fell in love with him. She realized he had probably been in love with her all along, just playing it cool so he wouldn't scare her.

Turning, Again, to Faith

At this time, since she had decided against reconstruction, Dana wore a prosthesis, which she hated. She was bothered by the way it felt and—much as she hated to admit it—by the way it looked.

It wasn't quite the same size as her natural right breast, so she couldn't wear her old bras. The only bras that were designed to support a prosthesis were old-lady-like and not attractive. Dana wanted to look pretty in her lingerie. Her clothing didn't fit the way it always had; she had to plan her outfit carefully every day. "I just don't want to work this hard so early in the morning," she complained to Jill. Besides, the prosthesis was heavy and its weight was a constant reminder of the cancer. She began to consider reconstruction. "When I can wear my bodysuit again, I'll know I'm all right," Dana told her parents.

And as she considered reconstruction, she began to worry about her other breast, and thought about her future health. After consultation with her doctors, she had some of her bone marrow harvested, because if the cancer recurred, she would be her own best donor. She was concerned about her other breast. After all, it too had received radiation treatment for Hodgkin's disease, so there was the risk of subsequent cancer in it as well. Throughout treatment, Dana asked her doctors about the risk of cancer in her right breast, but never felt like she got a straight answer.

After spending eight months in thoughtful discussions about the physical and psychological impact, Dana decided on a prophylactic mastectomy of her right breast. "It was a matter of knowing that, God forbid, should I get cancer again, I did everything I could," Dana said. "I'd rather not have the breast and be alive, than still have it and be worrying constantly." Her breast surgeon and oncologist agreed immediately. But it was still a difficult decision. For Dana, her right breast was sexual. When she lost her it, she would have no feeling at all in her breasts. She felt she was losing part of her sexuality.

Saying Goodbye

Again, Dana turned to Judaism for support. This time, she chose the *havdalah* ceremony, the Saturday night ritual that separates Shabbat—the Jewish Sabbath, which is a special and holy time—from the rest of the week. Havdalah literally means "separation;" Jews are sad at the closing of the special Sabbath day and the return to the ordinary week. The havdalah ceremony is an opportunity to focus on, and regret, that loss and separation.

Dana chose to do this ceremony privately, with Adam. "You've seen my body in every stage," she explained when she invited him to participate in the special havdalah ceremony. "You've seen me with two breasts, with one breast, and pretty soon you're going to see me with none."

They performed the ceremony naked from the waist up, in Dana's living room just after sunset on Saturday night.

Adam began. "A legend tells us that as night descended from the end of the world's first Shabbat, Adam and Eve feared and wept. Then God showed them how to make fire and by its light and warmth to dispel the darkness and its terrors. Kindling flame is the symbol of our first labor on the earth. Shabbat departs and the workweek resumes."

Then Dana spoke about her own separation, her difficult journey, and the beginning of the next piece of her life. Pointing to the blue-and-white twisted havdalah candle that Adam held, she spoke of "the light within" giving her strength, both physical and emotional. She spoke of the unforeseen blessings that she found in her illness: the people she met, the support she received.

Lifting the traditional silver spice box, Dana talked about the consoling quality of the fragrant spices. Saying the blessing over the kiddush cup, and taking a sip, she mentioned the way that "wine gladdens the heart."

At the end of the ceremony, after dousing the havdalah candle in the wine, Dana and Adam sang the traditional Shabbat song, "Shavuah Tov"—a good week, a week of peace.

Building a New Life

That July, Dana had her right breast removed and immediate reconstruction of both breasts, using tissue expansion and saline implants. It turned out that taking off the right breast was a good idea; the pathology laboratory found tissue that looked as though it might become cancerous.

The plastic surgeon put the tissue expanders in and it took about seven months to stretch her skin. During the tissue expansion, Dana began to dress normally again, although she felt like she'd had a watermelon on her chest for the past three months. She bought new bras for her somewhat expanded chest. "This size wasn't by choice," she explained to Adam. And, finally, triumphantly, she put on her bodysuit. "That means I'm okay," she told her mother with a grateful sigh.

After the surgeon inserted the permanent implants and Dana had nipple reconstruction, a plastic surgery nurse specialist tattooed on the areola.

As Dana began feeling better, she started to put in additional hours at work. Her director realized how much she had been doing and went to the board, petitioning them to make Dana full time, and threatening to leave herself if they didn't.

Dana was hired full time at the center, and over the next year and a half she became more and more involved in her work. She realized that she enjoyed working with healthy college students more than the more emotionally charged challenge of helping very ill children. She tried to find balance in her life between work time and play time. Working at Hillel allowed her to make a positive contribution in a way that didn't compromise her health.

Dana and Adam began talking about getting married and about Dana moving to Chicago. Dana found their relationship healing and felt good about making plans for the future. Through her connections in Milwaukee, she was able to secure a job at the Hillel center in Chicago.

Finding Meaning

Throughout her diagnosis and treatment for breast cancer, Dana never said, "Why me?" She was depressed, she was sad, worried, tearful, and sometimes angry. But she was never angry at God. "I never asked 'why me?' but rather, 'why did God choose me?' That is a different question," she said. "It's a question of finding the meaning in the experience, not self-pity."

As she told her brother Richie, "As awful as it was, my life would be so different if I didn't go through this. I wouldn't have such a good idea of who I am. I wouldn't have these close personal and family relationships. I wouldn't be married to this wonderful man. I wouldn't have realized all of these blessings. I wouldn't wish it on anyone, but I don't know if I'd change it, either. Because I just wouldn't be the same person, I wouldn't be Dana."

When Dana works with college students, she encourages them to think about breast cancer and other types of cancer. She has a sticker on her wall that reads "Fight Breast Cancer," because she *wants* people to ask her about it. She wants college students to know that she was *their* age when she was first diagnosed with cancer. She also wants women and men to know that they can talk to her about it. Dana loves what she does and believes it's really important to do something that is an extension of herself, that she gets something out of, that she truly enjoys.

Dana feels grateful that she's here, and she and Adam have an unusual awareness of the preciousness of each moment. They have adopted a son, Herschel. They try to do things now and not wait "for later." Dana realizes that it's important to enjoy the present.

Dana says, "Sometimes I really wonder if the 'reason' I got cancer was because I was supposed to adopt Herschey. That he was our *besheret* [Hebrew for "meant to be"] baby. We can have children biologically, but we choose not to because of the risk. We would have never tried to adopt a baby if my situation was different. Sometimes I really feel like it was a master plan—getting sick, meeting Adam, and finding Herschey—because we were meant to be together. This is what it all means to me now."

She returns often to the rituals of Judaism for comfort and thanksgiving. She finds herself saying a lot of *shechechiyanus*, blessings that she's happy to be here and to enjoy the moment.

*Baruch atta adonai elohenu melekh haolam shehehiyanu
vikiyemanu vihigiyanu lazman hazeh.* Blessed art Thou,
O Lord our God, King of the universe, Who have kept us
alive, and sustained us, and enabled us to reach this season.

*Dana and Adam are married and live in Milwaukee. They are working on
adopting a second child. Dana has been in remission for eight years and
is planning a blowout, over-the-top, everyone-she-loves-there, live-life-
fully party for her tenth year of remission.*

☐ ☐ ☐

Dana brought an unusual combination of research, creativity, and
religious ritual to saying goodbye to her breasts. Having family and
friends surround her and be involved in the ceremonies was particularly meaningful to her.

While no one else in this volume used religion in quite the same
way, Dana was lucky to be able to draw on her spiritual foundations
to help her come to terms with her new body. Not everyone has that
resource to draw upon.

CAN FAITH HELP WITH UNCERTAINTY?

✺ Robin, 33: Finding Faith in All Things

TALL AND SLENDER, WEARING A KNEE-LENGTH black leather coat,
black slacks, and leather boots, thirty-three-year-old Robin was possibly the best-dressed medical editor in Cambridge, Massachusetts.
Using her PhD in medical anthropology, she worked with physicians
to develop patient-friendly protocols for a high-end website. She was
responsible for putting together the epilepsy and breast cancer protocols. "If I'd worked on the testicular cancer protocol," she joked with

colleagues after her experiences with breast cancer and epilepsy, "maybe things would have turned out differently."

In 1999, Robin had buried her best friend, Mirel, who had died of leukemia. She had met Mirel, who was from Turkey, when they attended an international high school together in France. They had moved apart geographically after graduation, but remained close, and visited each other as often as they could. When Mirel was diagnosed with acute lymphocytic leukemia, Robin kept in close contact with her, visiting her in the hospital in Houston. For months, while she was in chemotherapy for the leukemia, Mirel would send Robin volumes about spirituality and illness, asking, "Could you read these and tell me if I should read them?" And Robin, being a good friend with an intellectual curiosity about spirituality, would read them. Some books she weeded out, others she recommended for Mirel, returning them to her in the hospital with comments and observations she thought her friend might find interesting.

Robin didn't practice religion herself, but she had respect for the concept of faith. She always thought of religion as a thread running through our daily lives. She thought that, perhaps, it would take on a more potent role under certain conditions, but she never really sat down to consider what those conditions might be.

꿏

A year after Mirel's death, Robin experienced her first grand mal seizure. She'd had smaller seizures for years, lasting no more than sixty to ninety seconds; these started when she was training in the martial arts in China and worked her body so hard that she stopped menstruating. The seizures never interfered with her life; when she'd mentioned it to her doctors, they never seemed concerned. But this experience was different.

Robin was meeting in her office with a coworker when she started to seize. Her face twitched, and she looked like she was in a trance.

The next thing Robin knew, she was lying on a bed in the emergency room and could feel a tugging on her eyebrow as the doctor stitched it. Her ex-boyfriend, Duke, a former NFL wide receiver, stood speechless and shocked in the corner.

The doctors conducted a slew of tests to rule out a brain tumor, determined that she'd had an epileptic seizure, and sent her home with anti-convulsion medication to prevent similar events.

Robin realized that her smaller seizures usually happened about a week and a half before she got her period. Could there be a hormonal cause? But her neurologist wasn't interested in discussing anything below the neck. She was having a bad reaction to her medication, too, and wondered whether she ought to find another doctor, one who could discuss her entire body. She made an appointment with a local internist who was highly recommended.

In the examining room, Robin began to enumerate her symptoms and describe her reaction to the anti-convulsion medication.

"Let's just start with a thorough checkup," said the doctor. When she got to the clinical breast exam, she felt a lump. "What is this?" the doctor asked.

Robin laughed. "My problem is in my brain, not my breast."

"I'd like you to get this checked out."

"I'm sure it's nothing. Doctors are always finding lumps in my breasts," said Robin. "Besides, I had a baseline mammogram three years ago, when I was thirty, and it showed nothing."

"Still," the doctor continued, "I'd like to get you in for a mammogram and an ultrasound."

The doctor set an appointment for the next day, but Robin was so unconcerned that she preferred to keep a lunch date with a good friend rather than do the tests immediately. A week later, the mammogram showed nothing and the sonogram—and the radiologist—confirmed Robin's opinion that her breasts were fine.

"This is a textbook picture of a benign lesion," said the radiologist. "Here's the tail, here's the curve," she said, pointing to the film as she spoke. "But because it's palpable, you really should see a surgeon for a biopsy."

Again, Robin had no anxiety about her breast; she was focused on resolving her seizures. She put the biopsy out of her mind until a coworker checked up on her.

"No, I haven't done it yet," said Robin. "I really don't think it's anything to worry about."

"Go get the biopsy," chimed in a radiologist colleague from down the hall. With a chorus of urging in her ears, Robin went back into her office.

Between her high-pressure job and the stress of trying to break off her seven-year relationship with Duke that just wouldn't go away, Robin didn't have time for what she thought was probably a pointless medical appointment. But she reluctantly made the appointment anyway.

Getting the News

When Robin went in for the examination, the breast surgeon took one look at the sonogram and confirmed what the radiologist had said, without a word of preamble. "It looks like a fibroadenoma." She proposed doing a fine-needle aspiration to test the lump. Initially, Robin had misgivings about the test, which was only about 85 percent sensitive. Even if it turned out negative, she would probably have to come back for a second procedure to make sure she was all right. But she agreed to have it done. The doctor performed the needle aspiration in a perfunctory manner. Finishing up, she turned to Robin on the table and said simply, "I'll get back to you on Tuesday." It was Thursday. Robin left the room without any further exchange.

That weekend, Robin went to Connecticut to visit friends. Saturday evening, Robin called home for her phone messages and was surprised to hear her surgeon's voice on the machine. She just left her name and said she'd call back on Monday.

Robin was simultaneously terrified and livid. What on earth could prompt the surgeon to call over the weekend, three days early? It simply wasn't fair to get her attention like that and then leave her hanging for another forty-eight hours. What was going on? She called the hospital immediately. Her surgeon wasn't in, but she could speak with the surgeon on call. "Fine," said Robin, indignantly. She figured she would insist that the surgeon on call connect her with her own surgeon.

Five minutes later, Robin's own doctor called. "It didn't come back as we had expected," she told Robin.

"You mean it was indeterminate? We have to do the test again?"

"No . . ." said the surgeon. "It came back as ductal carcinoma. You have cancer."

"In situ?" asked Robin incredulously, hoping for a contained cancer.

"You know the difference?" the surgeon asked.

"Yes, I know the difference," said Robin, annoyed at the way the surgeon underestimated her medical knowledge.

"No, it's invasive."

Robin started to dry heave. "Am I going to be able to have children?" she whispered.

"I didn't know you wanted any," said the doctor.

Robin was stunned. She didn't realize she'd been thinking about having children; the sentence that popped out of her mouth was a complete surprise. But at the same time, she didn't understand how a surgeon could assess her maternal instincts after having no conversation with her and respond to her so icily.

"Come to my office on Monday and we'll talk about next steps," the surgeon continued, then hung up.

Robin called her sister, Wendy, eighteen months her junior. Wendy worked at the American College of Obstetricians and Gynecologists in Washington, D.C., and was well connected in women's health issues. In addition, Wendy's husband was a surgeon at Georgetown University, so she knew a little bit about the topic. When she heard about the situation, Wendy decided to fly up to Boston to go to the appointment with Robin. On Monday morning, Robin and Wendy went to see the breast surgeon together. The conversation, as always, was brief. They set an appointment for a lumpectomy a week later.

Feeling a Failure

Robin was busy as she waited for the week to pass. She went back to work for a few days, slightly dazed but somehow able to focus on her job. On Thursday, she left for North Carolina to see her parents, a visit planned long before the biopsy.

The plane ride down wasn't much better than the train ride back to Boston. Robin knew she was bringing her parents a great sadness and she felt like such a failure. She'd always been the overachiever, the child who brought home A's and academic awards. But now she wasn't such a success. She had failed to save Mirel's life, had failed to revive her relationship with her boyfriend, failed to turn her doctoral dissertation into a book. And to top it all off, now she was coming home with cancer. She kept trying to script the conversation in her head, but couldn't come up with the right phrasing. I just don't see how I can do this, she thought.

Her parents took Robin to their favorite Vietnamese restaurant. Robin had always been very close with her mother; they were practically best friends. But she often clashed with her father. Somehow, though, this lunch was completely pleasant, one of the most peaceful meals they'd had together in a long time.

As they got back into the car to return to her parents' house, Robin's dad, Jimmy, said, "So, whatever happened about that biopsy?" They remembered that she had canceled the appointment to attend her grandfather's funeral.

"We got some results back, but we need to look at it a little closer to figure out what's going on."

Robin's mother, Ann, understood; she'd done the diagnostic dance with her own breast cancer diagnosis several years earlier. But Jimmy wanted more information. "Certainly they must have said something. They took out cells, what did they see?"

Robin took off her seat belt, slid into the center of the backseat, and put her head between the two front seats. "It's ductal carcinoma," she said.

The car was silent. Ann just stared at the highway. "How much?" she finally asked.

Robin couldn't bring herself to say the word "invasive." She just said, "They'll know more when they go in next week."

Ann lifted up her left hand and held Robin's right as they rode the rest of the way home, listening to the whirring of wheels on asphalt.

The rest of the weekend was very quiet. The three of them went for walks and ate at nice restaurants. Every night, Robin crawled in bed with her mother for an hour or two while her dad sat in an easy chair in the bedroom. Robin kept thinking about how difficult this must be for her parents. Parents are supposed to get the life-threatening diseases, not children. It was easier to focus on them, to think about their sadness, than to dwell on her own fears.

Robin was never very good at taking care of herself. She tried; she exercised a lot and ate a low-fat diet. But she overdid it. She dieted so much that she stopped menstruating; that was when the seizures started. Nor was she very good at taking care of herself emotionally; she protected the relationship with Duke more than she looked out for her own interests.

Duke flew back to see her. Robin had told him that she didn't expect him to stay with her through this experience. What she didn't say was that she would actually prefer he not stay with her. She knew her tendency to try to save the relationship above all else and worried that she would spend all of her energy trying to figure out how to make the relationship work, rather than focusing on taking care of herself. If Duke came back, she wanted it to be for good, to get married, not just to hang around for nine months of treatment.

When he arrived, Duke said that he thought she wanted him to come back and be by her side through treatment. If he came back, she wanted him to come back emotionally: to commit to a lifetime with her. She tried to explain the difference when he showed up on her doorstep, but he just said, "No, I'm staying."

Learning to Pray

Not long after Mirel died, Robin had received a strange package from Turkey. Mirel's parents had sent her the spirituality books she had screened for Mirel when she got sick. They thought their daughter's close friend would want them and perhaps take comfort from them as a reminder of Mirel.

Mirel and Robin had discovered the role of prayer together during her sickness, Robin remembered. After Mirel got back some encouraging test results, they went to the hospital chapel and sat quietly. But words of prayer had not yet come to Robin. And now all those books were here in Robin's living room. Robin piled them up in the corner of her desk, near the clinical literature that she so often perused.

⁂

The following week, Robin was in fine spirits on her way to the lumpectomy. Her mother, Wendy, and Duke were all there to offer support. Before the lumpectomy, the radiologist detected another possible lesion underneath the nipple. Robin asked whether the lesion should be biopsied at the same time as the original lump. After all, Robin knew, the lumpectomy would leave scar tissue and make it more difficult to find the second lump on film down the road.

"No, we'll deal with that later," said the surgeon curtly.

That made Robin nervous, but she didn't feel she had any other choices at the time. She hoped it would turn out okay.

When Robin woke up from surgery, the doctor had results for her. The sentinel node biopsy came back negative, which meant that the cancer had probably not spread to her lymph nodes and to the rest of her body. That was wonderful news, but the margins were not clean. She would need another lumpectomy, to be sure they got all the cancer. They scheduled the next surgery.

In the meantime, Robin met with the oncologist. "I would like to avoid chemotherapy, to protect my ovaries, if I can," she explained.

"I think that's reasonable," said the oncologist, "since your lymph nodes were negative."

Robin was thrilled. She, Wendy, and Duke went out to celebrate that night with a boat ride around the Boston harbor. "I may lose a breast," said Robin, "but my ovaries are going to stay intact."

The next day, Robin's training as a medical editor kicked in. Wendy, too, recommended she get a second opinion before deciding not to do chemotherapy. "My husband has a colleague at a hospital right here in Boston. He's not taking new patients, but just say you want a consult about whether you should do chemo." So Robin made an appointment with the doctor Wendy recommended.

When the appointment rolled around, Robin's mother and Duke went with her. As she sat in the room, a resident walked in.

"We've taken a look at everything you've sent us. Our strong recommendation is that you get chemotherapy," the resident began.

"Why do you have such a different view than my doctor at the other hospital?" Robin asked, concerned that she was speaking with a resident, rather than the doctor Wendy had sent her to see.

"Well," the resident began, "given your age and the fact that your lymph node was positive—"

Robin cut her off: "No, no, no. My lymph node was *negative*. That is very important. My lymph node was *negative*."

The resident looked down. Robin assumed she was taking a moment to compose herself for having made such a big mistake. Then she looked Robin in the eye and continued. "That's what I'm actually working myself up to tell you. They read your pathology reports wrong. Not only are your lymph nodes positive, but you have lymphatic vascular invasion that they completely missed."

Robin gasped. Her prognosis had just taken a major turn for the worse. And she knew it. She became incensed at the resident, who then left the room in search of the oncologist.

Robin was angry, angry, angry—*really* angry. She'd accepted that she had breast cancer. She was dealing with the diagnosis. And now she was being told that her chances of survival were much lower than she'd thought, that she would definitely need chemotherapy.

Then the oncologist walked in, having been briefed on the situation.

Robin started in with her questions. "What is this, some kind of Rorschach inkblot test, where one person can interpret the results one way and another can interpret it another?"

"The results are clear," began the oncologist. "It's a micrometastasis. It goes without saying that I am perfectly happy to take you on as a patient, given what has happened."

That's when Robin started to think, again, about prayer.

A Multifaceted Spirituality

One reason Robin never prayed was that, being a writer and a perfectionist, she could never find the right words. Any words she came up with always seemed so inadequate to the task she thought prayer was supposed to accomplish.

But when she was diagnosed with cancer, with invasive cancer, words started coming to her and she found herself in conversation with God from time to time. "Help me realize my blessings, help me realize the powers you've given me and really do something with them," she would say.

Robin knew some people might think the change was a psychological need, a conversation with herself. But she felt it was more than that. It went beyond a philosophical curiosity about God and religion or a response to extreme circumstances. It felt potent, like an authentic grasp of something extremely powerful that defines us as human beings.

Robin became particularly interested in the writing of Thomas Merton. She wished she could find a way to combine Catholicism, the mystery of God and faith and unknowable, with Buddhism. She was strongly drawn to the Buddhist philosophy of life and its attitude toward uncertainty.

While she classified herself as a Catholic, Robin found she was not comfortable with the word "religion," feeling that it had very limiting connotations. She preferred the word "faith." She didn't feel that her faith deepened; it wasn't so much a straightforward belief system, a simple round ball that looks the same from all sides. Rather, it was more like a Rubik's Cube, with myriad configurations and perspectives.

More Conflicting Advice

When Robin went in for her second lumpectomy at the second hospital, having fired the surgeon and staff from the first, the radiologist was skeptical that he would be able to find the lesion under the nipple to prepare it for biopsy. "Tell me the truth," Robin asked, "should the doctor have biopsied that at the same time she did the first?"

"Yes," he said, without hesitation. "It's going to be difficult to find now, with the scar tissue from the first lumpectomy." Using an MRI, though, he found it.

Robin just couldn't believe it. Both her pathology report and her surgery were messed up. "I'm a medical editor with a sister who can navigate any health system and a brother-in-law who's a surgeon," she told Wendy, "and these things still slipped through the cracks. What do people do who don't have my education and my kind of backup? How do they negotiate the human error that's so rampant?"

The surgeon performed the second lumpectomy, took out the second lesion, and did a full auxiliary node dissection, removing fifteen lymph nodes. The good news was that all the other lymph nodes were fine; the bad news was that the margins were still not clean. The cancer was larger than anyone had anticipated. At this point, the only alternative left was mastectomy.

Around this time, Robin and Duke started to look into fertility issues. With six good years and two bad ones behind them, they decided to harvest eggs before Robin had chemotherapy. Robin began taking Lupron injections and preparing to raise her estrogen level to make it easier to harvest a lot of eggs at once. Planning fertility was a bright spot for Robin and Duke, something positive they could focus on during a difficult time. And when Robin told her oncology resident, there was no objection.

When the lead oncologist found out what she was doing, however, he warned her against it. "Your cancer is very estrogen-receptor-positive, which means that estrogen encourages the cancer to grow faster. Raising your estrogen is *not* a good idea for you." Robin stopped the process.

Robin decided she wanted immediate reconstruction, so she had to pick a plastic surgeon and a method of reconstruction. She met with the doctor her oncologist recommended and felt very comfortable with him. When he recommended a latissimus dorsal flap, using skin and muscle from her back, she trusted his advice. She liked how he examined her and how he explained the pluses and minuses of each option. She decided to go with his suggestion.

Seeking Solace

The night after surgery, Robin felt like a loosely threaded piece of fabric. The surgeons had removed her breast and tunneled all of the muscle and nerve from her back under her arm and up over the implant, using about two hundred and fifty stitches. She just lay there, trying to keep as still as possible. It was reassuring to know her mother was sleeping on a cot down the hall.

When Robin was feeling her worst but was unable to speak for fear she'd rip apart at the seams of her stitches, a nurse came in and sensed her anxiety. She spoke softly of things Robin can no longer remember. She was very reassuring. The nurse stayed with Robin all night, until her shift ended in the early morning.

The doctors gave Robin about four weeks to recuperate from surgery before starting chemotherapy. Robin tried to prepare herself for what she knew would be a very difficult year of treatment and recovery.

The night before her first chemotherapy treatment, Robin made a visit to a Catholic church in Harvard Square. She usually didn't go to church—she had major disagreements with the Catholic Church's politics—but she didn't want to go home. She just wanted to be alone. The church was empty save for someone practicing the pipe organ. The music was spiritual and soothing.

Robin was in too much pain to sit up after the long walk to the church, so she just reclined on a wooden pew near the back and stared up at the three-story vaulted ceiling. She started to talk to God.

I don't want this chemotherapy tomorrow. You've got to help me find some peace with what I'm about to go through because I so badly don't want it. And I've been fortunate; I've never had to do anything I didn't want to do, except bury Mirel.

She just lay there, staring up at the ceiling, waiting.

Duke accompanied her to the first chemo session. When the nurse went to put in the first infusion, Robin just started crying. "I don't want this, I don't want this shit in my body," she said. "I know how toxic it is." She was sad, she was angry, and the tears were streaming down her face. She thought about how she'd gone with Mirel to so many chemotherapy infusions, and how unbelievable it was that she was doing it herself only a year and a half later.

Duke turned to the nurse and asked, "Why is she crying?"

The nurse just said, "Sometimes that's what people do." Robin was impressed by the simplicity—and accuracy—of the response.

After four months, Robin started to experience menopausal-like symptoms. Nurses and doctors kept telling her that her period would never come back, that she would just have to accept this change in her body. But her oncologist told her, "I'm placing my wager on your ovaries, Robin. Your body has a way of deciding what it's going to do and I think your period is going to come back."

Faith and Science

Even while Robin dreaded chemotherapy, even while she detested what it did to her body and her mind, she knew she was taking it for cultural reasons as much as for medical ones. She knew that the treatment offered her no guarantees. The data on chemotherapy's effect on survival rates was murky at best.

She realized that we have traditions for illness, as for health. And that one of those traditions is that when you get cancer, you have chemotherapy. She asked herself why she was doing chemo. And she recognized that she was taking a leap of faith. She didn't know that it was absolutely going to extend her life, she didn't have a rational reason for doing it. In fact, she decided, there was every reason in the world *not* to do chemo.

But Robin decided that she wanted to do *something* and she decided to place her faith in medical doctors. But, of course, she would continue to scrutinize and reflect on everything they told her; she would continue to make conscious choices about what to do. At her last chemo session, the oncologist said, "I guarantee that the cancer is not coming back."

Robin was very touched. For a doctor to step beyond the scientist, to give a guarantee, was a statement of faith. "This was the best gift he could give me," Robin told Wendy. "He's sending me out into the world with such a faith in me. It really means the world to me."

But Robin's relationship with her doctors was not all smooth. She ran into difficulties with the resident. The resident made a number of mistakes, in particular, failing to wash her hands before examining Robin, a grave concern for a chemotherapy patient who has a compromised immune system. In addition, she was very unfriendly, curt to the point of being uncompassionate.

Robin had been talking with a friend who came to her chemo about her concerns over the resident's failure to wash her hands. A nurse overheard the conversation and asked the name of the resident. Robin told her. That Friday, late in the afternoon on a snowy January day, Robin called to find out the results of her blood work. The resident gave her the results and then said, "By the way, you are no longer my patient."

Robin was confused. The resident was firing her? "Excuse me?"

"Let's just say that you seem really dissatisfied with my care," said the resident. "You are no longer my patient."

"I'm sick as a dog and we're heading into the weekend!" said Robin, thinking about how the resident had been her major point of contact at the hospital for three months now. "Who do I call if I have a problem?"

"Just call the hospital switchboard; they'll connect you with someone."

Instead, Robin phoned the oncologist, livid. "Let me tell you what this woman has done," she began. "I put up with this mistake of hers, and that mistake of hers, and now she fires me on a Friday afternoon when I'm sick as a dog."

"Sometimes patients and doctors have bad chemistry," the doctor began.

Robin cut him off. "This isn't about bad chemistry! It's about bad doctoring!"

The oncologist gave Robin his home phone and suggested she call over the weekend. They talked for hours, as Robin related her history with the resident. Finally, the oncologist said, "You're going to be my personal patient, I'm not going to pass you off to any other resident."

Robin was relieved. She knew that from this moment on, she would have the best possible care.

Discovering the Depths of Faith

One day, in an argument with Duke, Robin told him, "That's between God and me."

Duke just laughed. Having been raised in an African American Methodist church, he had always felt he had a stronger sense of faith than Robin and had always lorded it over her. Indeed, she'd often told him she wished she had grown up in such a church, where she might have gotten a better feel for faith.

"What do you know about God?" asked Duke. "You don't have any faith."

"That just shows what you know about me, about what I've been through," answered Robin. As she heard the words leave her mouth, she realized that, indeed, faith *had* been the backdrop and the infrastructure of her life, as she started to rebuild her life and her sense of self-care. It wasn't until she told Duke that she realized how much she had changed.

Chemotherapy Aftermath

A year after Robin finished chemotherapy, her period came back. She called her oncologist and told him, "You win. It came back."

He wasn't surprised.

But menstruation was a mixed blessing. Within a week of getting her period, she had three small seizures and slipped into what she could only describe as total cellular fatigue. She was so tired she couldn't move for twenty days out of the month. She had just moved to New York to work for a nonprofit and found that she couldn't make it into the office. Fortunately, the organization was very flexible and arranged for Robin to do her job from home. So, she would get up, work for half an hour, roll back into bed for a few hours, then get up and work a little more. Moreover, her whole body was in pain, from her feet to her brain stem; she could barely hold her head up. Doctors had no idea what was going on. They thought maybe it was arthritis, maybe she had lupus or chronic fatigue syndrome. But the symptoms and diagnosis never jibed.

At Robin's one-year checkup with her oncologist, she asked, "How did this stuff affect my endocrine system, which I think is messed up and which is why every other system is messed up?"

The oncologist sat on a stool with wheels. He pushed himself back across the room, crossed his arms across his chest, and said, "It's nothing we did to you."

Robin was disappointed; for the first time, she felt her oncologist had let her down. His body language said he thought she was accusing him of some kind of wrongdoing. She knew he responded as he did because he wanted her to feel well, to be well, and that it was painful not to have an explanation, much less a solution, for her fatigue and pain.

A New Faith, Rewarded

Robin's next-door neighbor, Cynthia, was knowledgeable about various types of alternative treatments. They became friendly and one afternoon Robin tried to explain her symptoms and her frustration.

"Nobody is providing any viable explanations for why I can't walk, move, breathe, open my eyes," she told Cynthia. Her muscles were tender, she couldn't walk, and she just felt pain, pain—pain in her neck, her feet, her back. Her feet, for instance, literally pulsed with pain; she could watch them throbbing.

"My medicine cabinet is just filled with painkillers and medication," Robin explained. "But they're not providing me any relief and they're very hard on my liver. Every morning, I wake up wondering how the chemotherapy is going to affect me today. And I feel so depressed. I mean, I paid the dues, I had my breast cut off, I had my ovaries reamed with chemicals. Why do I have to keep paying the price?"

"Maybe your body can handle the normal estrogens, but it might help to limit the environmental estrogens, the stuff like plastics and pesticides that act like estrogen in the body," Cynthia suggested. "Maybe you should look into enzymes for detoxification."

Cynthia's suggestion made a lot of sense to Robin and she started researching. "The problem with this stuff is that it has not been very well researched, and what research was done is not very well documented," she told Cynthia. "I find I have to read and read and read. I have to check cross-references and multiple sources of information. I have to read as critically as when I was deciding between a lumpectomy and radiation or a mastectomy."

She began taking enzymes and ended up taking more than a dozen supplements daily. "But I'm only on two prescription drugs—at half the dose I used to take. And I'm a thousand percent improved," Robin said triumphantly. "While traditional medicine obviously has enormous benefits, it also has enormous limitations that bear directly on young women and breast cancer. Traditional medicine has no clue how chemotherapy affects our endocrine system, how it affects the pituitary glands, the hypothalamus, and how all those organs communicate with our ovaries."

When Robin went to see her oncologist, she explained, "I'm my own clinical trial," handing him a list of everything she was taking. "Here's my list of medicines and magic potions," she told him. "I call them 'magic potions' because I know that's what you think they are. I'd like you to look at it and comment on anything that looks obviously wrong."

"To be honest, at this point you know more about this stuff than I do," the oncologist said. "I trust your judgment."

Complementary Therapy

The supplements continued to work. In April, Robin had twelve functional days; in May, she had eighteen. She started thinking, if she

---

Survivor Suggestions on Alternative Therapies

The women in this book have benefited from a variety of alternative or complementary therapies during and after their breast cancer treatment. They include:

- acupuncture

- affirmation tapes

- alterations in diet; macrobiotics; vegetarianism

- art therapy

- Ki energy therapy

- massage

- meditation

- psychotherapy

- reiki

- visualization

- vitamins and/or enzyme supplements

- yoga

could just get it up to twenty good days, that would be all the work days in a month.

Robin decided that she needed to get back to exercising. She began with yoga classes, then included weight lifting and extensive cardio exercise as well. She was always careful to take it slow and wear the dual sports bra her plastic surgeon recommended, to help prevent the breast implant from exploding. She thinks that the rule about avoiding repetitive movements and lifting weights isn't universally applicable. Most women recovering from breast cancer, Robin figures, would probably benefit from exercise. Doctors told Robin she would never regain feeling on the right side of her back, but she has definitely regained a little bit of feeling. It seemed to her that if you build muscle, you're going to build nerve, you're going to build blood flow, and you're going to build feeling.

Reflections on Spirituality

"I have found that there's a very short distance between religion and science," Robin says. "They are first cousins. And I approach faith and religion with a healthy skepticism, just as I do doctors' orders. And I approach my doctors acknowledging that I am placing a certain amount of faith in them, as I do in a person of the cloth.

"To the extent that cancer and especially its treatment are transformative, that has to affect you spiritually. I just don't know how it can't. That doesn't mean it has to deepen your faith, but it will give you pause to reflect on everything around you in a way that you didn't before," she said. "And to me, that is fundamentally a spiritual experience."

Robin is still working as a medical researcher in New York City. She is four years out from her diagnosis and is doing well, although she experiences hormonal fluctuations and their side effects. The herbal and nutritional supplements continue to help her tremendously.

　　　□ □ □

Through her experiences with breast cancer, Robin reevaluated her relationship with God and religion. She was far from alone in this response. After hearing the diagnosis, Barbara and Dawn's husband found themselves angry with God, while Robin, Dawn, and Dana felt a stronger relationship with God. "I'd always been devoutly agnostic," Nora told her mother. "I thought this experience would help me make a decision. I figured I would either know God existed or didn't." But she ended up just as questioning as ever, if a little irritated at her continued agnosticism.

In addition, Robin explored prayer and, through her experiences, found words with which to pray. Dana, too, developed her relationship with prayer. Unlike Robin, she did not create a vocabulary for prayer where there had been none; rather, she adapted and expanded her existing prayers and rituals to meet her new needs. For Robin, Dana, and Dawn, breast cancer strengthened their connection to religion and religion helped them handle the disease, its treatment, and aftermath. Their faith was a source of solace and understanding.

CAN FAITH DEEPEN?

⚜ Dawn, 31: A New Relationship with Jesus

AT AGE THIRTY-ONE, DAWN WAS A BUSY WOMAN. She juggled her family responsibilities, her waitressing job at a family restaurant, and college, where she had just started a course to become a physical therapy assistant. She'd only been married to Mitch, her second husband, for about eighteen months, and she had two children.

Her son, Anthony, age nine, was dealing with developmental depression and had already tried to commit suicide three times. He was an emotional roller coaster, swinging from deep depression to worrisome violence. He had recently gone to live with his father, who lived about two hours away, in hopes that a change of environment would help.

Tiffany, thirteen, who lived with Dawn and Mitch, was blossoming into a lovely young woman. She was an A student and helped out cheerfully at home. Dawn was very proud of how mature Tiffany was becoming.

Dawn had been a practicing Catholic all her life. The whole family went to church on Sundays, the children attended catechism, and they had a crucifix in the living room. All four pretty much agreed on the important role of Catholicism in their lives. Dawn didn't set out looking for a deeper relationship with Jesus. It came to her.

Questioning Fate

One Saturday morning, about a month after she had gone back to school, Dawn felt a lump in her right breast while she was changing shirts. She mentioned it to Mitch, who told her not to worry, but to be sure to call the doctor first thing Monday.

She did, and the doctor saw her immediately and sent her for a mammogram. The morning after the mammogram, she got a call telling her to schedule a biopsy. Now she was really getting nervous. She wanted to get in for that biopsy as soon as possible. She had a bad feeling about all this.

But the recommended surgeon couldn't make an appointment for more than a week. Dawn worried that this was too long to wait, so she called the local cancer research institute and found a doctor there to fit her in the following Monday.

"I'm sure this is nothing," said Mitch, upbeat, as he rescheduled his day at the tool-and-die shop to attend the appointment with Dawn. "You had a full physical exam just a few months ago and your breasts were fine."

"I don't know," Dawn said slowly. "I have a feeling it's cancer." Mitch just shook his head.

They walked into the examining room together. Dawn sat on the examination table and Mitch perched himself in a chair facing her while the doctor performed the biopsy. "We should have the results back on Wednesday," said the doctor. "But let's make the appointment for Thursday in case the lab is late."

It was a nervous few days for Dawn. She kept turning the possibilities over in her mind; she was sure she had cancer, but still didn't want to hear the definitive diagnosis. She was glad she'd gone with the cancer institute. As long as this wait felt, she would have an answer before she could even have laid eyes on the surgeon her doctor had recommended.

On Thursday, Dawn and Mitch came back and sat waiting in the room for the doctor. She walked in and said, "Well, it looks like we have a little cancer."

Mitch went white and he sat very still. "I knew for sure you didn't have it," he whispered.

"I knew for sure I did," said Dawn just as quietly. The consequences of the diagnosis didn't really occur to Dawn at that moment; she just saw how pale and vulnerable her husband looked.

She sat there, hands in her lap, and thought about her family. Her mother had been struggling with ovarian cancer and chemotherapy treatment for several years. Her aunt had been diagnosed with breast cancer earlier that year.

Then it hit her. She had nothing planned. Who would take care of her children if something were to happen to her? How would her daughter function without a mother? And what about her son, who was already suffering from developmental depression?

"How could it happen to you?" asked Mitch. "You're the kindest person. You're always helping people. You care about everyone."

"That doesn't matter, Mitch," said Dawn.

"There are so many really bad people out there," he continued. "How come *they're* not sick?"

Dawn never questioned why it happened to her. She never worried specifically about dying, only about not being around for her children. But Mitch was much more troubled. He began to doubt his belief in God, and stopped going to church altogether.

Dawn, too, sought answers. But she searched within religion, within her belief in God's power to heal and to give answers.

People Deserve Better

Mitch went to every appointment with Dawn. They went together to the plastic surgeon, oncologist, and breast surgeon. He attended every chemotherapy treatment. He was always right there in the room with her.

Dawn had her surgery on a Friday in October. Because her cancer was so aggressive—both breasts had checked out just fine three months earlier—she agreed to undergo a bilateral mastectomy, just in case. It turned out that her left breast was cancer free. She chose TRAM flap reconstruction for both breasts. The surgery took eleven and a half hours—longer than expected, but Dawn's plastic surgeon was a meticulous and dedicated perfectionist.

It was late at night when Dawn came out of surgery. The hospital staff allowed the whole family, about fifteen people, into the recovery room. Dawn was woozy and white as a ghost. Anthony walked right up to his mother, took her hand, and stroked her wrist. Dawn was awake enough to know he was speaking to her, although she couldn't process the words he was saying.

Tiffany had a harder time of it. She just stared at her mother and started to cry. Dawn's sister hugged her from behind as Tiffany continued to watch her mother through her tears.

Dawn was in the hospital for five days and felt that the nursing care she received left much to be desired. "I have to wait a long time for things to get done after I buzz the nurses," she complained to Mitch. "I kept calling the nurse to empty my fluid, and it got full to the top."

"And you were in bed for three days before anyone got you up to try walking," Mitch added, worriedly.

"People deserve better than that," said Dawn.

Dawn was released from the hospital on Wednesday and took the rest of the week off. She went back to school the following Monday, having missed only one week of classes. She still had four drains in place when she went back to school, so she wore button-down shirts to hide them. "I can hear my drains swishing as I walk down the hall," she told Mitch, feeling both embarrassed and amused. Chemotherapy and school were about all she could handle, so she quit her waitressing job. The people at her restaurant were very understanding and begged her to keep in touch.

Dawn started chemotherapy at the end of the month. When she went to see the oncologist, she was excited that she was going to lose weight and told the doctor that. The oncologist looked at her like she was crazy.

"You're not going to lose weight, you're going to gain weight. The medicine you're going to get will make you crave protein; you're going to want huge steak-and-potato meals. And while you will probably be nauseated, most women find that chewing makes them feel better."

Dawn lost all her hair after the first treatment. It was already very cold in Michigan and Dawn found that she preferred hats to wigs. Both she and her husband kept their sense of humor about it all.

"Hey, why don't we paint your head orange and put you out on the porch for Halloween?" Mitch suggested.

They joked that Dawn might be too tired to play on the billiards team, but she could be the mascot. "We could paint your head black and put a white '8' on it," Mitch suggested.

Watching the Children

Hearing her parents joking about breast cancer made it easier for Tiffany to handle her mother's illness. She'd always been mature for her age, she'd lived through her grandmother's illness, and she just didn't seem as scared as one might expect a child her age to be. Tiffany felt comfortable asking her mother all sorts of questions about breast cancer and treatment, and came to know when Dawn was having a bad day. She asked about Dawn's hair loss, fatigue, crankiness, and her prognosis. Dawn was careful to answer only the questions Tiffany asked and to try not to scare her daughter. She was pleased she could be open with Tiffany, who seemed to take everything—from fatigue to baldness—in stride.

"You're having to grow up a little sooner than I would have liked," Dawn told her. "But I am very proud of how mature you've become." Dawn hoped she wasn't keeping everything inside.

As it turned out, it was a good thing that Anthony was living with his father at this point. "We certainly couldn't take care of him now," Mitch commented. "And he might have felt like he was being punished if we sent him away when you were diagnosed."

"It was also good for me, to give me time to get used to him not being here. I really think it's taken me a year to adjust. It's good to know that he's being taken care of, to know that he's doing well in school and at home. I really do miss him. But, you know, I think God had it planned out perfectly," said Dawn. "He knew I was going to be sick in a year, and He knew that we needed Anthony to be healthy. And He knew that we both needed to be at peace with him not living here."

"Salvation Is a Gift from God"

As she dealt with her cancer, Dawn started searching spiritually. She had a new hunger for spiritual food and now had more time to explore and ask questions.

She worried about what would happen when she died. "Because I'm right there—I have a life-threatening disease. I could die," she explained to Mitch. Dawn started reading and talking to people of different faiths, looking for answers.

She began talking to her neighbor Debbie, a born-again Christian. Dawn had always thought she was a bit "far-out" in her religious beliefs. But as they talked, Dawn became intrigued by Debbie's Bible-based faith.

"In Catholicism, in order to go to Heaven, you do whatever the pope has decreed. But for those who are born again, you go to your salvation, heaven, which is a gift of grace from God. All you need is faith."

"That's what people often find so refreshing about being born again," said Debbie. "You don't have to perform works for grace, it is a gift from God."

To learn more, Dawn and Mitch took a class at Debbie's house. They read the Bible and other books written about Jesus as Messiah. Dawn grew to appreciate this new view of salvation, which she found more meaningful than what was taught in the Catholic church.

Dawn also became friendly with a young woman named Tina, who listened carefully to Dawn's questions about religion and offered answers that were never pushy. Just by being a "kindred spirit," by praying with Dawn and attending church with her, Tina was instrumental in nurturing Dawn's growing faith. She also became a close friend.

As Dawn continued to study through the class, both with Tina and on her own, she decided to leave the Catholic church. She decided to step over the line of faith, to put her faith in Jesus, to become born again. She joined Debbie's nondenominational church. That was how she wanted to live her life.

"Now I'm just as far-out as my neighbor," she told Mitch with a smile.

"Yep, you're just a Holy Roller," Mitch joked back.

Cancer in the Genes

By Christmas Day, most of the family's women were bald. Dawn, her aunt, and her mother all sat around the dinner table wearing various head coverings: Dawn wore a hat while her aunt and mother preferred wigs. After dinner, Dawn and her sisters worked on a greeting card for their father, who lived in Iowa. They drew a Christmas tree on Dawn's head with green face paint, wrote "Merry Christmas" underneath, and took a picture of it.

Dawn's mother and aunt started exploring the family's history of breast and ovarian cancer. They discovered that Dawn's maternal grandmother and great-grandmother both had died of ovarian cancer. Several cousins had died of breast cancer. And now Dawn and her aunt had breast cancer.

Encouraged and led by Dawn's mother and aunt, the family got involved in a medical study about the BRCA1 gene, the first gene known to predispose women to breast cancer. Everyone in the family was tested and it was determined that Dawn does have it. Another of Dawn's three sisters also has the breast cancer gene. Dawn burst into tears. "I can't say I'm surprised," she told Mitch. "I've already had the disease; I figured I had the gene." Having the gene in *her* body wasn't what upset her. It was her children. "This means that I could possibly pass the gene on to my kids."

The doctor told her that because she was part of the study, her children could be tested for the gene, if they chose, when they turned eighteen.

Progress and Setbacks

Dawn finished chemotherapy in April, and followed up with the remainder of her reconstruction surgery, including nipples and a tattooed areola. Soon after she finished chemo, Dawn developed strange symptoms. Her tongue and ankles swelled up, and she lost much of her ability to remember things, to think straight, and to concentrate. She didn't want to see the doctor until after her upcoming physical therapy certification exam, so she just struggled on, finding it harder and harder to study and retain information. On the day of the exam, Dawn was exhausted and having trouble thinking straight, but she got through it. The minute she got home, however, she called her doctor for an appointment.

Blood work determined that Dawn had hypothyroidism, an illness that typically afflicts older women who have undergone radiation treatments. Her thyroid levels were so low that she should have been in a coma. She was given medication and felt its effect within days. Her thoughts were clearer and her memory returned.

She was not surprised to learn that she failed her exam and flunked out of the physical therapy program. But with typical energy and resilience, Dawn immediately began thinking about what she wanted to do next. She remembered the poor nursing care she had received when she was in the hospital and decided that perhaps nursing would be a better fit for her. She registered for nursing classes, to begin the coming fall semester.

Staying Ahead of the Gene

In July, Dawn's mother died, ending her seven-year struggle with ovarian cancer. The BRCA1 gene predicts not only breast cancer but also ovarian cancer. Indeed, doctors told Dawn that she had a 45 to 50 percent chance of getting ovarian cancer. A month after her mother's death, Dawn had her ovaries removed prophylactically. She figured that she'd already had her children, and she wanted to be around to take care of them. The BRCA1 gene also increases her chances of colon cancer, though to a much lesser degree than breast or ovarian cancer. So just to be safe, Dawn has a colonoscopy every two years.

"It has to be your decision whether to get tested for the BRCA1 gene," Dawn told her daughter. She was more direct with Mitch. She told him that she hoped Tiffany would choose to have the test done. "I want her to be tested because if she has the gene, I would want her to do everything prophylactically that she can. And if she needs to make decisions about starting a family, I want her to have that information, that choice," said Dawn. "I want her to have prophylactic mastectomies and once she has her children, I want her to have her ovaries removed."

Timing was key. Doctors told Dawn that since she had the gene, her children should be screened ten years earlier than she was when she got diagnosed. "My mom was forty-five when she found her lump and I was thirty-one," she said.

"So that means Tiff should be followed starting at age twenty-one," Mitch said.

When she turned eighteen, Tiffany decided to be tested for the gene. The day they went for the blood work results, Dawn was terrified at the possibility of having passed the gene on to her daughter. But Tiffany was completely calm. "If I don't have the gene, then praise God. And if I do have it, God's going to use that somehow, God's going to use that in my life."

Dawn was impressed by the extent of Tiffany's faith. She realized that her daughter had seen the way breast cancer had brought positive changes to her own life. Tiffany's understanding of her mother's experience only strengthened her own faith in God and in His plan.

To the family's immense relief, Tiffany tested negative for the breast cancer gene.

Respecting Spiritual Change

Dawn's faith affected her family as well. She was reintroduced to God and introduced to a new relationship with Jesus through her cancer. She witnessed to her family and now her children live that life, they live for God. Dawn was very proud of them.

Mitch hasn't moved in the same spiritual direction as Dawn. While he was respectful of her beliefs, he didn't share them. He held hands as they prayed before dinner, but sat silently, and only occasionally attended church with the family. Dawn prayed every day that he would come to know God the way she had. But she understood that her disease caused him to question his faith. Although she might not understand why he made the decision he did, Dawn was as respectful of Mitch's choices as he was of hers.

Mitch thinks that Dawn is no longer the woman he married. "You changed when you became born again," he said, looking around the house, with wooden crosses and little painted signs reading *Jesus Is the Way*.

"No, I haven't," Dawn protested. "You have to remember, not only am I a born-again Christian now, but I'm a woman who's survived cancer, who's been through chemotherapy, who's had five image-altering surgeries. My shape is completely different and I have scars that I wouldn't want anyone to see," she explained. "I went through so many different emotions, so many changes in self-image, so much pain. How could I *not* be changed by all that?"

Dawn still feels the effects of her disease and treatment. She has started seeing a chiropractor because of pain in her stomach and back, due to the surgery and chemotherapy. "You think it's over, seven years later," Dawn says. "But it's not. I still have no feeling in my breasts—I never will. I have no abdominal strength, because of the reconstruction surgery. And I gained forty-five pounds because of the chemo."

Dawn set new goals for herself. "I'm not yet forty years old, but I'm looking forward to forty being the best. By forty, I want to look and feel the best I've ever been. I have a new career now. I have stronger faith. I want to get back to my pre-chemo weight. I don't know if I would have had the ambition to do all these things if I hadn't had cancer."

And she is on her way. She has recently joined Weight Watchers and lost fifteen pounds right away.

Seeing Blessings in Breast Cancer

Dawn is now a labor and delivery nurse. "Without breast cancer, I would have settled for being a physical therapy assistant, which is a great career and helps a lot of people. But being a nurse takes me one step further. I have opportunities as a nurse to work with so many different people. I can work in the community, I can work in hospitals, I can work in oncology, I can work with children, I can work in labor and delivery." And her experience with breast cancer is a gift to her as a nurse. "I know how people feel who are in pain or are scared. I can honestly tell them I know how they feel. Because I've been there."

"I'm stronger and more confident than I thought. If I could get through that, I could pretty much get through anything. That's what the whole year brought to me."

Dawn considers breast cancer a great blessing in her life, one of the best things that's ever happened to her. She was reintroduced to God and introduced to Jesus. She's gained inner strength and inner peace. She's met people through diagnosis and treatment. "When you go through a crisis like breast cancer, it shapes your relationships. They're either going to be strengthened or they're going to fall apart." Her faith deepened and her relationship with Jesus became a great comfort to her. And her relationships with Mitch and with the children are stronger than ever before.

Dawn is still happily married to Mitch. Anthony, a high school senior, is healthy and has decided that he will probably be tested for the BRCA1 gene when he turns eighteen. Tiffany graduated from college with her mother in attendance and was married in the spring of 2004.

□ □ □

Dawn used religion as a way to seek answers about how to live her life and turned to Jesus to find those answers. But while she is unusual in the questions she investigated, she is not alone in exploring philosophical questions. Amanda asked why she, who'd always followed the rules, was hit with the disease; Jacquie wondered why teenagers could bring children into the world while she, who was so much more prepared emotionally and financially, could not. Helen wondered how to make a difference in the world, and Susan worried about what qualified as "acceptable risk" for herself and a potential child.

Most women, like Dawn, read and talked with people to explore their concerns. Susan filled a two-drawer file cabinet with pertinent academic and magazine articles and was accused of "consultativitis" because she spoke with so many physicians and researchers.

For Dawn, faith was the answer. But that wasn't true for everyone. Jacquie, for instance, specifically chose not to talk with her mother about her diagnosis because she did not want to be told to put her faith in God. Similarly, some women felt the way Dawn's husband, Mitch, did; they became angry with God. Mitch had a spiritual crisis, stopped going to church, and broke off his relationship with religion.

Nora, too, found that breast cancer prompted questioning about a higher being. She had always been agnostic, but thought that the life-threatening experience of having breast cancer would help her find God. She felt that she would either come to know that God existed, or decide that He didn't. In the end, she was no clearer on the issue than she'd been before, which she found frustrating.

Faith does not help everyone. But when questions are unknowable, God and religion can often provide a reassuring answer that gives you a structure to move on.

ॐ

Religion—and God—can become a pivotal focus during difficult or transitional periods. Some get angry with God. Some people question; Amanda wanted to know why she was chosen to have breast cancer when she had always "followed the rules," and Nora became frustrated that she didn't come to understand God as a result of her disease. Barbara was very angry with God and demanded of Him: "Why is this happening to me? I thought you were supposed to watch out for good people!" She even began to wonder, "What kind of a person am I to have something so devastating happen?" Conversely, others, such as Dana, Robin, and Dawn, found comfort and meaning in religion, faith, spirituality, and God.

But there are many ways to turn to religion and many forms of religion to turn to. Some people emphasize ritual, traditional actions associated with religion. They find great meaning and comfort in activities such as going to synagogue or church or having a ceremony of some sort. For Dawn, going to church was important; for her husband, ceasing his attendance expressed his attitude toward God and religion. For Dana, the process of creating rituals to say goodbye to her breasts was very meaningful.

Other people turn to spirituality for answers to emotional searches. Dawn found that becoming a born-again Christian helped her understand how she should lead her life. Religion helped her understand her emotional response to the disease.

Spirituality can also address philosophical concerns, providing a framework for thinking about the unknown, the unknowable. Robin found, in a less formal spiritual approach, a way to rethink her life after breast cancer, which was, in itself, a spiritual undertaking.

Indeed, if you subscribe to Robin's attitude about spirituality, everyone in this book has altered her life as a result of the experience with breast cancer. Some women have changed their careers or work-life balance; some have rethought how—and whether—to date; several have reconsidered bearing or adopting children; they have changed their attitudes toward religion; and almost everyone has become more politically or socially active.

No woman can face a life-threatening disease without rethinking her life, without reassessing her decisions and striving to control her life. In this way, every woman who has breast cancer is transformed in some way, whether overtly religious or not.

Survivor Suggestions on Faith, Religion, and Spirituality

- Approach breast cancer treatment as a journey.

- Embrace the joys of life.

- Don't take things or people for granted.

- Learn to accept uncertainty.

- Don't ask "why me?" but look for meaning in the experience.

- Realize your blessings and your own power. Celebrate them both.

- Keep your sense of humor.

- Consider using religious rituals as a source of strength: to say goodbye to a breast or hello to a new body. It can be a creative and meaningful outlet for strong emotions. Allow others to become involved in rituals that you create, to enable them to help and show their concern in a meaningful way.

- Let breast cancer make you more open to thinking about God and spirituality. And realize that the experience will not affect everyone the same way. Respect others' decisions the way you hope they will appreciate yours.

- Realize that cancer and its treatment may give you pause to reflect on everything around you in a way that you didn't before.

Life After Breast Cancer

Life begins anew when a young woman comes out on the other side of breast cancer and its treatment. Even if her day-to-day routine returns to normal, she is, invariably, a changed person. Whether the change is physical, emotional, spiritual, or some combination thereof, life after breast cancer is much different from life before it.

THE WOMEN WHOSE STORIES are contained in these pages have grown tremendously as a result of their experiences with breast cancer. They have realigned their priorities in terms of work, friends, and "self-care," to use Robin's term. They have reevaluated their relationships with their own bodies and reconsidered their ideas about having children. They have gained personal insight and recognized their inner strength. And they have become more socially and politically active. Many young women say they emerge from the breast cancer battle with greater sensitivity, confidence, and strength.

When Nora was first diagnosed, a friend and breast cancer survivor told her that she would get something out of the experience of having breast cancer. Nora retorted, "Like fuck I will." But when she looks back on the experience, Nora realizes she was wrong. Having breast cancer did change her perspective on her life by helping her rethink her priorities and enhance her self-awareness.

241

As Dana explains, "I never asked 'why me?' but rather 'why did God choose me?' That is a different question. It's a question of finding meaning in the experience, not of self-pity."

Other women explored similarly philosophical questions. Dawn thought about how best to live her life each day and how to prepare for the possibility of death. Helen wondered how to make a difference in the world, looking for a place where she could leave her mark. Susan worried not about *risk*, but about *acceptable risk* for herself and for the child she wanted to have.

For Dawn, faith was the answer to a life-threatening disease. Similarly, breast cancer gave Dana a way to come to terms with her new body. It provided Robin with a scaffold for reconstructing her life.

Robin believes that no woman can face life-threatening disease without rethinking her life; thus every woman who has had breast cancer is transformed in some way. "To the extent that cancer and especially its treatment is transformative, it has to affect you spiritually. I just don't know how it can't."

INCREASED ACTIVISM

Many young women who have had breast cancer become more politically and socially active as a result of their experiences with the disease. Several of the women profiled in this book, for instance, became involved in raising research money for and social awareness about breast cancer.

Some started their own organizations. Roberta and Lanita were two of the founders of the Young Survival Coalition and Susan helped found its Massachusetts/Rhode Island chapter. Mary started Rocky Mountain Team Survivor, an activity-focused alternative to the standard support group, and Janis is a founding member of Silent Spring Institute, which funds research into the environmental causes of cancer in general.

Others work for existing organizations. Janis is also active in fundraising for the Massachusetts Breast Cancer Coalition. Barbara flew to Washington D.C., with her doctor to testify before Congress about the importance of breast implants. Paulette and her daughter, Claire, run together in the Susan G. Komen Race for the Cure.

Just about everyone I interviewed informally counsels other young women with the disease, particularly those who have been recently diagnosed. A common thread in the counseling they give is the importance of performing monthly breast self-examinations. As Janis explains, "That's how I found my lump." Indeed, most of the women in this book found their lumps and brought them to the attention of their physicians.

REALIGNED PRIORITIES

Many breast cancer survivors realign their priorities in a variety of ways as a result of their illness. Some rethink their careers and the long hours they put into their jobs. Others begin to think differently about unfulfilling friendships. Some change their ideas about sexuality, dating, and family. Some have learned to give themselves permission to be more self-indulgent. And some simply change their overall perspective on life.

Many women switch careers after having breast cancer. Helen, for instance, moved from law to professional advocacy. Often, additional education is required for such a move; Helen was lucky because she already held a master's degree in public administration, the pertinent degree. Barbara, however, went back to school to get her high school diploma and take some college courses, which allowed her to move off the factory assembly line into medical office work. Dawn completed high school, went on to nursing school, and is now a labor and delivery nurse. Jacquie changed course from an MBA to a doctoral program and now works in university administration.

Roberta, Mary, and Janis all decided that they enjoyed their careers, but wanted to adjust the balance between their work and the rest of their lives. They all cut back on their workweeks. The once-workaholic Roberta now takes weekends off, much to her colleagues' surprise. Mary elected to work part-time to allow more time for herself. Janis switched jobs to a position with more regular hours.

Dana became more firmly ensconced in her career choice, working with college students until she adopted her son. Similarly, Anne became more committed to continuing her education and landing her dream job.

Dating is another area affected by having breast cancer. Becky and Dana stopped dating during treatment. Becky felt more fragile and vulnerable; she was less willing to trust and more afraid of making the commitment necessary to a long-term relationship. Both eventually came to terms with their fears and are now married.

But Anne, even after finishing treatment, had a rough time. "The problem with breast cancer and relationships is that things move more quickly physically than they do emotionally," she says. When Anne was diagnosed with cancer in her bones and lungs, she stopped dating altogether.

Much of this feeling of rejection stems from adjusting to a changed body. Breasts carry tremendous symbolic value in terms of both sexuality and motherhood. And it is not only the disease itself, but even treatment that can hurt a woman's self-image. Scarring from surgery, reddened and tender skin from radiation, and weakness from chemotherapy significantly affect a woman's physical self-confidence. Thus, even the most confident and self-assured women find it hard to feel desirable and lovable when their bodies are so radically affected by cancer treatment.

Reconstruction can help women regain a sense of themselves as a whole. For Amanda, Dana, and Barbara, breast reconstruction after mastectomy was a critical part of reclaiming their sexuality and getting back to their normal lives. But not everyone feels that way. Mary, for instance, worried about the side effects of reconstruction and sees her mastectomy scar as a badge of honor that in itself instills confidence and pride. "Having my breast removed, having the mastectomy, made me a better warrior in a sense," Mary said.

Breast cancer causes some women to rethink whether—and how—they want to have children. Jacquie, who was pregnant when she discovered her lump, found she couldn't have children after treatment; she would have to adopt. Dana and Helen also decided to adopt, because of concerns over their own health. Lanita adopted because of her concerns over passing on increased risk.

Susan, Amanda, and Roberta all decided to give birth, after being reassured that medically it was a reasonably safe option for them. For Susan, this was a particularly dramatic decision, as she became a single mother when Diana was born.

Nora made changes in her friendships, deciding to eliminate the "bullshit" of the film world. Helen, too, lost some friendships during treatment. Dawn agreed that relationships are often changed by breast cancer. "When you go through a crisis like breast cancer, it shapes your relationships. They're either going to be strengthened or they're going to fall apart." She was lucky; her relationships with family and friends were fortified through her experience.

Similarly, Janis tried to make more time for people who are important to her. She decided that her relationships with friends and with her parents are more significant than working a little harder. Roberta agreed. "Before, when people invited me to events I would often say, 'Oh, I'm so busy.' But after breast cancer, I say, 'I wouldn't miss it for the world.'"

Some women tried to take better care of themselves. Janis, for instance, stopped smoking. Nora started standing up for herself, which is not to suggest that she became less caring. "It's very important to me to be a good person," she said. "If I die five years from now—and I do have a one in five chance of being dead five years from now—I don't want to feel regrets. I want to live my life so that when I die, I'll know I did the best I could."

Barbara tried to take particular care of her children as well. When her daughter Brooke turned seventeen, she began smoking cigarettes. "You are responsible for the choices you make in life," she told Brooke, who ultimately quit.

GREATER SELF-AWARENESS

Successfully battling breast cancer also bestows greater self-aware-ness and increased confidence on younger women. Janis, for instance, felt a greater awareness of her own drive and vitality. "I have come to believe that we're only as strong as the circumstances we're dealt. And that we don't realize our strength until we're put in a situation that tests it. Then we find the inner strength we need."

Susan found a new understanding of the concept of risk. "Up until breast cancer, I never thought of myself as being seriously 'at risk' for any major health issues. I never had to make decisions like, 'Do I take a drug that will increase my risk of one cancer in order to decrease my risk of another cancer?' When life starts to look like that, you realize that you're living in a world of risks."

Paulette looked at having the breast cancer gene in that same way, as something that you must accept and move on from. "People have con-trol over some things," she said. "You can control what you eat, how you vote. But some things, like breast cancer, are just handed to you."

Greater self-awareness can also mean some melancholy. Dana, for instance, worried a lot about getting sick again. Janis allowed that there is a new sadness in her, too. She was not sure whether it stemmed from her experience with breast cancer or from something else. But she had come to realize that perhaps it's not so important to pin it down. She used her sadness to fuel her activism. And Jacquie still makes love in the dark.

But most of all, these women talk about positive changes coming from their experiences with breast cancer. Anne explained, "If any-thing, fighting cancer has made me *more* confident and strong." Dana explained, "As awful as it was, my life would be so different if I hadn't gone through this. I wouldn't have such a good idea of who I am. I wouldn't have developed these close relationships. I wouldn't be mar-ried to this wonderful man. I wouldn't have realized all of these bless-ings. I wouldn't wish breast cancer on anyone, but I don't know if I'd change it—having had breast cancer—either. Because I wouldn't be the same person. I wouldn't be Dana."

The sixteen women in this book, as well as many others I spoke with, used their experiences with breast cancer as opportunities to rethink their lives and to find power within themselves. They made changes in their careers, families, friendships, spirituality, and many other areas they hadn't expected breast cancer to affect. These changes bring them greater fulfillment, joy, and pride in themselves than they had before.

These women are not just muddling through their days; they are actively deciding how they want to live their lives. These faces of breast cancer are not demoralized and depleted; they are vibrant, dynamic, brimming with promise, and full of life.

Survivor Suggestions and Thoughts
on Breast Cancer in General

☐ After you've had a biopsy, don't just sit around and wait for the diagnosis; go out and do something.

☐ Know that life will get better. It may not be a straight arrow shooting upward, and there may be bumps in the road, but it will improve.

☐ Don't see breast cancer as a less-serious disease because it mostly strikes women.

☐ Don't be ashamed of having breast cancer.

☐ Remember that cancer happens to good people, too. It is not a failing and it isn't your fault.

☐ View chemotherapy as "healing juice." But be prepared for its physical and emotional effects.

☐ Allow daily living—as well as physical therapy—to get you back into shape.

☐ If surviving cancer means maintaining some of your pre-cancer life, do it. For instance, don't shy away from bars just because you can't have alcohol; sip soda or a cup of coffee.

☐ Realize that the end of treatment may not be a time of festivity. Think carefully about planning a party or big celebration.

☐ Do breast self-exams. And encourage friends and relatives to do them as well.

Glossary

AXILLARY LYMPH NODE DISSECTION: Surgery to remove lymph nodes from the armpit area.

BIOPSY: Removing cells or tissues to check under a microscope. There are three kinds of biopsy: incisional biopsy or core biopsy, in which only a sample of tissue is removed; needle biopsy or fine-needle aspiration, in which a sample of tissue or fluid is removed with a needle; and excisional biopsy, in which a whole tumor or lesion is removed.

CHEMOTHERAPY: Treatment with drugs that kill cancer cells or make them less active.

Unless otherwise noted, all definitions are courtesy of www.breastcancer.org. If you would like to learn how to pronounce these words, or would like to see additional terms related to breast cancer, go to www.breastcancer.org and click on the Celebrity Talking Dictionary.

DUCTAL CARCINOMA IN SITU (DCIS): Abnormal breast cells that involve only the lining of a milk duct. These cells have not spread outside the duct into the normal surrounding breast tissue.

ESTROGEN-RECEPTOR-POSITIVE (ER 1): Breast cancer cells that have a protein receptor molecule that binds to estrogens. Breast cancer cells that are ER 1 depend on the estrogen hormone to grow. Anti-estrogen hormone therapy blocks the cancer cells' receptors and typically causes the cancer cells to shrink or die.

FIBROADENOMA: A benign (noncancerous) tumor. Fibroadenoma is the most common benign tumor of the breast and the most common breast tumor in women younger than thirty. Fibroadenomas are usually found as solitary lumps, but about 10 to 15 percent of women have multiple lumps that may affect both breasts.*

FINE-NEEDLE ASPIRATION: A test that uses a hollow needle to remove tissue or fluid. Then the material is looked at under a microscope to see if it is normal or abnormal.

IMPLANT: A manufactured sac that is filled with silicone gel (a synthetic material) or saline (sterile saltwater). The sac is surgically inserted to increase breast size or restore the contour of a breast after mastectomy.**

INFUSAPORT: A metal disc placed under the skin that is able to withstand multiple needle punctures and is often used for drawing blood or administering chemotherapy

LUMPECTOMY: Surgery to remove cancerous cells and a small amount of normal tissue around them.

---

*MedlinePlus, http://www.nlm.nih.gov/medlineplus, a service of the National Library of Medicine and the National Institutes of Health.
**Hyperdictionary's medical dictionary: www.hyperdictionary.com.

LYMPHEDEMA: A condition in which too much lymph fluid collects in tissue. This causes swelling. It can happen in the arm after lymph nodes in the underarm are removed. It can also happen if there is radiation to the lymph nodes or chemotherapy. It can get worse if the arm is hurt in any way.

LYMPH NODE: A rounded mass of lymphatic tissue that is surrounded by a covering of connective tissue. Also known as a lymph gland. Lymph nodes are spread out along lymphatic vessels and contain many lymphocytes, and act as a filter system for the lymphatic fluid (lymph).

MAGNETIC RESONANCE IMAGING (MRI): A test that looks at areas inside your body. Detailed pictures are made by a magnet linked to a computer. These are read by a radiologist.

MAMMOGRAM: An X-ray picture of the breast.

MASTECTOMY: Surgery that removes the whole breast.

METASTASIS: The spread of cancer from one part of the body to another.

METASTASIZE: To spread from one part of the body to another.

PAGET'S DISEASE: A type of breast cancer that involves the nipple. The cancer cells start in the milk ducts at the surface of the nipple. As the cancer grows on top of the nipple, it forms a dry, crusty, bumpy rash. It can cause itching and burning around the nipple. Sometimes it can also cause oozing or bleeding. Some doctors might think it is just eczema or dry skin. But if you have these changes, and they don't go away, be sure to see a breast specialist.

PROPHYLACTIC MASTECTOMY: Surgery to remove one or both breasts in order to reduce the risk of developing breast cancer. Also called preventive mastectomy.

RADIATION: The use of high-energy radiation from X-rays, gamma rays, neutrons, and other sources to kill cancer cells and shrink tumors. Radiation may come from a machine outside the body (external-beam radiation therapy), or it may come from radioactive material placed in the body in the area near cancer cells (internal radiation therapy, implant radiation, or brachytherapy). Systemic radiation therapy uses a radioactive substance, such as a radiolabeled monoclonal antibody, that circulates throughout the body. Also called radiotherapy.

RADICAL MASTECTOMY: Surgery for breast cancer in which the breast, chest muscles, and all of the lymph nodes under the arm are removed. For many years, this was the most common operation for breast cancer. It is rarely performed today.

RECONSTRUCTION: Rebuilding or repairing an area of the body that has been damaged or removed.

SENTINEL (LYMPH) NODE BIOPSY: Procedure in which a dye or radioactive substance is injected near the cancer and flows into the sentinel lymph node(s), the first lymph node(s) that cancer cells are likely to spread to from the main cancer. A surgeon then looks for the dye or uses a scanner to find the sentinel lymph node(s) and removes it (or them) to check for the presence of cancer cells.

SONOGRAM: Also called ultrasonogram or ultrasound. A test that uses sound waves to create images of structures within the body. The pictures appear on a computer screen. They can also be put on film.
stage I breast cancer: Cancer that is no bigger than 2 centimeters (about 1 inch) and has not spread outside the breast.

STAGE II BREAST CANCER: Stage II breast cancer means one of the following:
 • cancer is no larger than 2 centimeters but has spread to the lymph nodes in the armpit (the axillary lymph nodes), or

- cancer is between 2 and 5 centimeters (from 1 to 2 inches) and may have spread to the lymph nodes in the armpit, or

- cancer is larger than 5 centimeters (larger than 2 inches) but has not spread to the lymph nodes in the armpit.

STAGE III BREAST CANCER: Stage III breast cancer is divided into stages IIIA and IIIB.
- STAGE IIIA BREAST CANCER is defined by either of the following: (1) the cancer is smaller than 5 centimeters and has spread to the lymph nodes under the arm, which have grown into each other or into other structures and are attached to them; (2) the cancer is larger than 5 centimeters and has spread to the lymph nodes under the arm.

- STAGE IIIB BREAST CANCER: Stage IIIB breast cancer is defined by either of the following: (1) the cancer has spread to tissues near the breast (skin, chest wall, including the ribs and the muscles in the chest); (2) the cancer has spread to lymph nodes inside the chest wall along the breast bone.

STAGE IV BREAST CANCER: Cancer has spread to other organs of the body, most often the bones, lungs, liver, or brain; or cancer has spread locally to the skin and lymph nodes inside the neck near the collarbone.

SUPPLEMENTAL SECURITY INCOME (SSI): A federal income supplement program funded by general tax revenues (not Social Security taxes). It is designed to help aged, blind, and disabled people who have little or no income, and provides cash to meet basic needs for food, clothing, and shelter.*

TAMOXIFEN: A drug used to fight breast cancer cells that have hormone receptors. It can reduce the risk of a new breast cancer. It can

*www.socialsecurity.org

also delay the return of breast cancer and control its spread. It blocks estrogen receptors on breast cancer cells. This can slow down or stop the growth of cancers that need estrogen to grow. It belongs to the family of drugs called "selective estrogen receptor modulators," or "SERMs."

TRAM FLAP PROCEDURE: TRAM stands for transverse rectus abdominus muscle, which is located in the lower abdomen. In most women there is enough skin, fat, and muscle here to reconstruct a new breast. The tissue can be detached and moved, or the tissue can remain attached as a flap and slid under the skin up to the chest. In either case, the tissue is sewn into place as a new breast. The excess skin and fat that are removed from the lower abdomen can be considered a "tummy tuck," which some women appreciate as a fringe benefit from the surgery.

ULTRASOUND: Also called sonogram. A test that uses sound waves to create images of structures within the body. The pictures appear on a computer screen. They can also be put on film.

VASCULAR LYMPHATIC INVASION: When cancer cells break out of the place where they started and go into the lymph and blood vessels inside the breast. This is how cancer cells can travel to other areas of the body.

Resources for Additional Information and Assistance

Throughout these stories, the women I interviewed reiterate the importance of building a support network and gathering information. Their resource suggestions are given below, and include a range of major organizations and websites available. Here are support organizations, research groups, and activist organizations, as well as groups geared specifically to African Americans, lesbians, Jews, and others. Web addresses and phone numbers, where available, are supplied, and most websites offer links to related organizations. Do bear in mind, though, that the vast majority of these organizations are *not* geared specifically to women ages forty and younger.

ADELPHI NEW YORK STATEWIDE BREAST CANCER HOTLINE & SUP-PORT PROGRAM is a nationwide, community-based, voluntary health organization that offers a hotline, support groups (including one focused on young women), writing workshops, and online technical information. (800) 877-8077; http://adelphi.edu/nysbreastcancer/aboutus.html.

AMERICAN BAR ASSOCIATION'S BREAST CANCER LEGAL ADVO-CACY INITIATIVE provides information on breast cancer in the law and helps survivors find local free legal help. (312) 988-5715; http://www.abanet.org/women/.

AMERICAN BREAST CANCER FOUNDATION provides free breast cancer screening services to women of all ages who cannot afford them. Women who qualify are placed with local Centers for Disease Control and Prevention breast and cervical cancer screening programs. Online information covers breast cancer and mammograms. (877) 539-2543; www.abcf.org.

AMERICAN CANCER SOCIETY provides information on cancer, early detection, treatment decision tools, clinical trials, complementary and alternative medicine, and coping. The ACS runs Reach to Recovery, which offers support and information either face-to-face or by phone. (800) ACS-2345; www.cancer.org.

AMERICAN INSTITUTE FOR CANCER RESEARCH is a national cancer charity focused on nutrition and cancer. It provides research and consumer education programs. (800) 843-8114 or (202) 328-7744; www.aicr.org.

AMERICAN SOCIETY OF CLINICAL ONCOLOGY (ASCO) helps patients find board-certified oncologists. (703) 299-0150; www.asco.org.

ASSOCIATION OF CANCER ONLINE RESOURCES, INC. is a searchable archive for cancer mailing lists. It also provides fact sheets on a range of topics. (212) 226-5525; www.acor.org.

AVON BREAST CANCER CRUSADE helps women without health insurance find free or low-cost mammograms in their area. Avon funds many groups to provide this service. (212) 244-5368; www.avon-breastcare.org.

BIG BAM! provides medical services to women who experience age, financial, or cultural barriers that prevent detection and treatment of breast cancer. It hosts free mammogram screenings and ensures follow-up treatment for underserved women diagnosed with the disease. (212) 595-6525; www.bigbam.com.

BOSTON'S CRUSADE AGAINST CANCER. Services include a mammography van, a peer-education program, and a community partnership that works to create a culturally competent system of prevention and care for women of African descent. (617) 534-9650; http://www.bphc.org.

BREAST CANCER ACTION is a political activism organization that works with policymakers in government and industry at the local, regional, and national levels. (415) 243-9301 or (877) 2STOPBC; www.bcaction.org.

BREAST CANCER FUND identifies and advocates for elimination of environmental and other preventable causes of the disease. (415) 346-8223; www.breastcancerfund.org.

BREAST CANCER RESOURCE COMMITTEE offers a breast cancer awareness campaign geared to the African American community. (202) 463-8040; http://www.afamerica.com/bcrc.

BREAST CANCER SITE is a website that offers the option of donating free mammograms or shopping at sponsoring merchant sites, with a portion of each purchase going toward the cause. www.thebreast-cancersite.com.

BREASTCANCER.NET is an online news service that offers breast cancer–related news, and links to organizations and sites of interest to breast cancer survivors. www.breastcancer.net.

BREASTCANCER.ORG provides information about breast cancer prevention, symptoms and diagnosis, treatment, recovery, and resources. Online resources include illustrations of how to do a breast self-exam, types of breast cancer, treatment, diagnosis, and breast anatomy. www.breastcancer.org.

CANCER CARE provides emotional support, information, and practical help to people with cancer and their loved ones. Services include on-site and telephone support groups and newsletters. www.cancer-care.org.

CANCER NEWS ON THE NET offers the latest news and information on cancer diagnosis, treatment, and prevention. www.cancernews.com.

CELEBRATING LIFE FOUNDATION promotes breast cancer awareness, targeting African American women and women of color. (800) 207-0992; http://celebratinglife.org/Foundation_Profile.htm.

COMMUNITY BREAST HEALTH PROJECT offers information, support, and resources. (650) 326-6686; www.cbhp.org.

COMPASSION IN DYING FEDERATION provides legal advocacy and public education to improve pain and symptom management, increase patient empowerment and self-determination, and expand end-of-life choices to include aid-in-dying for terminally ill, mentally competent adults. (503) 221-9556; www.compassionindying.org.

FINDCANCEREXPERTS.COM helps patients get a second pathology opinion anywhere in the country. Fax: (301) 231-4987; www.findcancerexperts.com.

FLORIDA BREAST CANCER COALITION is a grassroots organization advocating for government funding for breast cancer research. (305) 669-0011 or (877) 644-FBCC; www.fbccoalition.org.

GEORGIA BREAST CANCER COALITION (GBCC) focuses on advocacy and legislative issues. Its sister organization, the Georgia Breast Cancer Coalition Fund (GBCCF), develops and promotes educational programming. (770) 452-7988; www.gabcc.org.

HURRICANE VOICES raises awareness, activity, and support in pursuit of the causes of and cures for breast cancer. (617) 928-3300 or (866) 667-3300; www.hurricanevoices.org.

IMAGINIS offers news and information on breast cancer prevention, screening, diagnosis, treatment, and related women's health topics. (404) 210-5922; www.imaginis.com.

LIVING BEYOND BREAST CANCER is committed to empowering women to take an active role in their recovery. Services include educational conferences, a resource center, and a Young Survivors Network. (610) 645-4567; www.lbbc.org. Survivors' helpline: (888) 753-5222.

MASSACHUSETTS BREAST CANCER COALITION focuses on activism, advocacy, and education. (617) 376-6222; www.mbcc.org.

MAUTNER PROJECT FOR LESBIANS WITH CANCER provides counseling and other services to lesbians with cancer and their partners. (202) 332-5536; www.mautnerproject.org/communty.html.

MOTHERS SUPPORTING DAUGHTERS WITH BREAST CANCER (MSDBC), a national nonprofit organization, provides free support services to mothers who have daughters battling breast cancer. (410) 778-1982; www.mothersdaughters.org.

NATIONAL BREAST CANCER COALITION (NBCC) is a grassroots effort that seeks to eradicate breast cancer through action and advocacy, focusing on research and access to care. (202) 296-7477 or (800) 622-2838; www.natlbcc.org.

NATIONAL CANCER INSTITUTE offers breast cancer care guidelines, statistics, and information on clinical trials. The International Cancer Center of the NCI offers news and abstracts from the *Journal of the National Cancer Institute* and other NCI publications, and CANCERLIT, an archive of more than a million bibliographic records describing cancer results published for the past thirty years in biomedical journals, proceedings of scientific meetings, books, technical reports, and other documents. (800) 422-6237; www.nci.nih.gov.

NATIONAL CENTER FOR COMPLEMENTARY AND ALTERNATIVE MEDICINE (NCCAM), an arm of the National Institutes of Health, supports rigorous research and disseminates information on complementary and alternative medicine. (888) 644-6226 or (301)519-3153; www.nccam.nih.gov.

NATIONAL COALITION FOR CANCER SURVIVORSHIP (NCCS) is a survivor-led advocacy organization that offers information and tools for survivors and caretakers. (301) 650-9127 or (877) 622-7937; www.canceradvocacy.org.

NATIONAL LIBRARY OF MEDICINE operates Medline, a database with more than fourteen million citations of research studies published in peer-reviewed, scientific journals. http://www.ncbi.nlm.nih.gov/PubMed.

NATIONAL LYMPHEDEMA NETWORK provides information on the prevention and management of primary and secondary lymphedema. (510) 208-3200 or (800) 541-3259; www.lymphnet.org.

ONCOLINK is an online resource that provides information on specific types of cancer, updates on cancer treatments, and news about research advances.www.oncolink.com.

1 IN 9: THE LONG ISLAND BREAST CANCER COALITION promotes awareness of breast cancer and other cancers through education, outreach, advocacy, and direct support of research.
(516) 357-9622; www.1in9.org.

ROCKY MOUNTAIN TEAM SURVIVOR is a health and fitness support group for cancer survivors. (303) 247-1212; www.rockymtn-teamsurvivor.org.

SHARE: SELF-HELP FOR WOMEN WITH BREAST OR OVARIAN CANCER helps people with breast or ovarian cancer to be more in control of their lives during and after diagnosis. (212) 719-0364; (888) 891-2392. Hotline: (212) 382-2111; www.sharecancersupport.org.

SHARSHERET connects young Jewish women recently diagnosed with breast cancer with volunteers who can share their experiences, both personal and medical. All conversations are confidential. (866) 474-2774; www.sharsheret.org.

SILENT SPRING INSTITUTE is a nonprofit scientific research organization dedicated to identifying links between the environment and women's health, especially breast cancer. It is a partnership of scientists, physicians, public health advocates, and community activists. (617) 332-4288; www.silentspring.org.

SISTERS NETWORK provides emotional and psychological support, resources for medical research, and community cancer prevention programs to African American women. (866) 781-1808; www.sistersnetworkinc.org.

SUSAN G. KOMEN FOUNDATION works through a network of U.S. and international affiliates to fund research, support education, screening, and treatment programs around the world. An online resource, www.breastcancerinfo.com, offers information on topics ranging from early detection to support. The foundation also sponsors the Komen Race for the Cure, the largest series of 5K runs/fitness walks in the world. (800) 462-9273; www.raceforthecure.com or www.komen.org.

SUSAN LOVE MD is a nonprofit organization dedicated to breast cancer education, research, and advocacy. The website offers information on reading a biopsy report, understanding treatment options, and choosing a doctor. www.susanlovemd.com.

ULMAN CANCER FUND FOR YOUNG ADULTS provides information, support groups, and college scholarships to young adults with cancer. www.ulmanfund.org.

VITAL OPTIONS INTERNATIONAL: SUPPORT FOR YOUNG ADULTS WITH CANCER is geared to young adults with cancer and provides cancer communications services including The Group Room radio show, a weekly syndicated cancer talk show that is simulcast on the World Wide Web and XM Satellite. This talk-radio program allows people from around the world to meet, talk, exchange information, and support one another. (800) 477-7666; www.vitaloptions.org.

WOMEN'S INFORMATION NETWORK AGAINST BREAST CANCER offers treatment information and peer support for patients throughout diagnosis, treatment, and recovery. (626) 332-2255 or (866) 2WIN-ABC; www.winabc.org.

Y-ME NATIONAL BREAST CANCER ORGANIZATION'S mission is to ensure, through information, empowerment and peer support, that no one faces breast cancer alone. Y-ME has the only twenty-four-hour hotline staffed entirely by trained breast cancer survivors. Additionally, eleven affiliates throughout the nation provide services such as support groups, early detection workshops, wigs and prostheses for women with limited resources, and advocacy on breast cancer–related policies in their respective communities. For breast cancer support or information, including publications and newsletters, visit www.y-me.org or call the Y-ME National Breast Cancer Hotline. (800) 221-2141 (English, with interpreters available in 150 languages) or (800) 986-9505 (Spanish).

Northern California affiliate: northerncalifornia@y-me.org

Southland California Affiliate: southlandcalifornia@y-me.org
website: www.y-me.org/southlandcalifornia

San Diego affiliate: sandiego@y-me.org

Rocky Mountain affiliate: rockymountain@y-me.org
website: www.y-me.org/rockymountain

Connecticut affiliate: connecticut@y-me.org

Illinois affiliate: illinois@y-me.org
website: www.y-me.org/illinois

Indiana affiliate: indiana@y-me.org

Northeastern Oklahoma Affiliate: northeasternoklahoma@y-me.org

Chattanooga Affiliate: chattanooga@y-me.org

National Capital Area Affiliate: nationalcapitalarea@y-me.org
website: www.y-me.org/nationalcapitalarea

Texas Gulf Coast Affiliate: texas@y-me.org
website: www.y-me.org/texasgulfcoast/

YOUNG SURVIVAL COALITION seeks to educate the medical, research, breast cancer, and legislative communities and to persuade them to address breast cancer in women forty and under through action, advocacy, and awareness. It also serves as a point of contact for young women living with breast cancer. www.youngsurvival.org.

Acknowledgments

SITTING DOWN AT THE KEYBOARD MAY BE A SOLITARY ACTIVITY, but writing a book is not. This volume could never have happened without the help of many people; my apologies, in advance, to anyone I forget to mention here.

First, I would like to thank all of the women who shared their stories with great patience, insight, compassion, and hope. This book is for you.

Thank you, thank you, to my editor, Molly Mullen Ward. You read my manuscript and immediately understood it. Then you helped guide it to become even closer to what it was meant to be. Thanks so much to my publicist, Lauren Lawson, for helping to share this vision with the world. And thank you to Paula Decker for stepping on the boat toward the end of the ride and seeing the project through to the end.

For helping me find women interested in sharing their stories, I must thank Calvin Allen, Susan Carr, Rose Day, Debra DeVitto Dunbar, Lynn Elliott, Lisette Garcia, Donna Kaye, Michelle Volpe Kluchman, Tom Mendolsohn, Merritt A. Mulman, Ann Palmer, Linda Rahijah, Gail Stein, Katherine Volk, Darcy Gammon Wakefield, Sue Ward-Diorio, and the Young Survival Coalition.

I am grateful to Bernie Hyman, Michael Stephens, DeWitt Henry, Osie Adelfang, and the folks at Emerson College for help in conceptualizing and developing the book. And I would like to thank Anne Fallucchi for a lifetime of mentoring and editing.

A special appreciation to Darcy, who read and reread every word of this manuscript for years and offered incisive comments, never-ending support, and a sun-shower of kind notes.

Thank you to my friends and cheerleaders, Debby Viveros and Lisa Brody Ritchie. You've been behind me every step of the way and I know how lucky I am to have you both.

Loving thanks to my intelligent, beautiful, and creative joys, Maya and Ari. You give me pleasure, insight, and a healthy distraction from my work. You are gifts beyond any I could ever hope for.

I am everlastingly grateful to Robert, who gave me the time and space to work on this book, perceptive comments on the writing and content, and love to make it all worthwhile. You believed in me when even I had doubts.

Any mistakes are, of course, my own.

Index

A